Macular
Degeneration

Macular Degeneration

THE LATEST SCIENTIFIC
DISCOVERIES AND TREATMENTS
FOR PRESERVING YOUR SIGHT

Robert D'Amato, M.D., Ph.D.,
AND
Joan Snyder

WALKER & COMPANY   NEW YORK

First published in the United States of America in 2000 by
Walker Publishing Company, Inc.

Medical disclaimer: The treatments and therapies described in this book are not intended to replace the services of a trained health professional. Your own physical condition and diagnosis may require specific modifications or precautions. Before undertaking any treatment or therapy, you should consult your physician or health care provider. Any application of the ideas, suggestions, and procedures set forth in this book are at the reader's discretion. Extreme caution should be observed when considering unproven, more invasive therapies that may adversely affect your health.

Library of Congress Cataloging-in-Publication Data

D'Amato, Robert.
    Macular degeneration : the latest scientific discoveries and treatments for preserving your sight / Robert D'Amato and Joan Snyder.
        p.   cm.
    Includes bibliographical references.
    ISBN 0-8027-1359-9
    1. Retinal degeneration—Popular works.   I. Snyder, Joan R.   II. Title.

RE661.D3 D36 2000
617.7'35—dc21

00-028991

Book design by M. J. DiMassi

Printed in Canada
2   4   6   8   10   9   7   5   3   1

CONTENTS

PART TWO
Treatment Options

PART THREE
Coping with Age-Related Macular Degeneration

ACKNOWLEDGMENTS

Without the help of several very special people, this book would not have been possible. Among them are Lisa Ross, whose idea for the book grew from both professional creativity and personal understanding; Nina Ryan, whose supportive input helped make it a reality; and Jackie Johnson, whose infinite patience and consideration enabled its production.

Many people with ARMD were also a continuing inspiration. Their personal candor with their experiences helped the authors understand the human dimension of this particular disease.

PREFACE

Robert J. D'Amato, M.D., Ph.D.

Many people have someone in their family affected with age-related macular degeneration (ARMD). ARMD is the leading cause of blindness in the United States and other developed Western countries. Approximately one third of the U.S. population over age sixty-five, or some 13 million seniors, have ARMD. My grandmother was afflicted with this disease, which robbed her of much of her vision in later life. My father also has early ARMD, but without serious vision loss to date. Although heredity is only one factor that determines a person's risk of developing ARMD, I do wonder about my fate. Like most people, I want to exercise some control of my health as I age and I hope to experience the most that life offers. This is one reason I work on treatments for ARMD. The other is the exhilarating, but sometimes exasperating, challenge of scientific discovery.

Because of my research on methods of stopping abnormal blood vessel growth, a feature of late ARMD, I was interviewed by ABC's *20/20* for a story on ARMD. After the show aired on TV, I was flooded with calls from patients throughout the United States. I was surprised to find that even patients who were far along in the course of ARMD had a very poor understanding of their disease process. How could a patient who has been to the doctor's office for laser treatment not understand that the treatment was attempting to destroy a blood vessel in his eye? Did the doctor not explain it fully, or was the patient unable to follow what was being said? The answer may be a bit of both.

It is very difficult to concentrate after a doctor has told you that you may lose your vision in an eye. Unfortunately, if your doctor has a busy medical practice, he or she may not be able to talk with you at length about your condition and make sure you understand it. Further, if you have preconceived notions about ARMD that are incorrect, they may interfere with your ability to absorb the information presented by your physician. The explanations and advice in *Macular Degeneration* are not meant to be prescriptive or to take the place of visiting your own medical professional. But it is my hope that by reading this book at your leisure, you will be able to make sense of ARMD and go to your next appointment ready to ask informed questions and participate fully in decisions about treatment.

At this writing, there is no cure for ARMD, but there are several research initiatives that may lead to better treatments or an eventual cure. Throughout history, many diseases affecting seniors have been attributed to the normal process of aging. Until the causes were understood, these diseases, such as Alzheimer's disease, were thought of as part of senile dementia or a progressive aging of the brain. As neuroanatomists discovered that specific areas of the brain were degenerating in Alzheimer's disease, in a pattern that was not part of normal aging, it became clear that this was a unique disease process which could be studied so that treatments could be developed. In a similar way, we now know that ARMD is a pathologic process with features that distinguish it from the normal aging of the retina.

Despite the overwhelming prevalence of ARMD, it has been one of the least studied diseases. Unfortunately in science, the squeaky wheel gets the grease. There has been very little publicity relating to ARMD, and advocates for the disease have gone unnoticed. Well-organized lobbies for diseases such as AIDS and breast cancer have led to tremendous advances in treatment. In ophthalmology, the gene for retinitis pigmentosa (RP)—a very rare eye disease—was recently discovered as a direct result of research sponsored by foundations and endowments supported by patients with RP. Finding the genetic abnormalities responsible for RP has unlocked a tremendous amount of research and provides a foundation for developing new treatments. The same level of research effort needs to be mounted for ARMD.

My purpose in writing this book is to assist patients in understanding the disease and potential treatment options as well as to raise public awareness about ARMD. When you have been diagnosed with macular degeneration, your first challenge is to gain enough technical knowledge to make informed decisions. Your immediate tasks are the following:

- Learn the vocabulary of the disease and the terminology that you will be hearing from the medical community.
- Understand the relative degree of severity for your particular condition.
- Familiarize yourself with the medical options for dealing with the degree and the type of macular degeneration you have.
- Stay up-to-date on pending treatments, clinical trials, or tests that are experimental or on the cutting edge.

I hope you find the material in this book helpful in reaching these goals.

PREFACE

Joan Snyder

My interest in assisting Dr. D'Amato with this book was twofold. As a person who has had age-related macular degeneration for several years, I was eager to help others understand the disease and learn how to manage it as effectively as possible, while representing firsthand the needs and concerns of someone living with ARMD. The second reason was more personal: I was searching for answers. It was my way of dealing with a diagnosis that came to me as shocking news from a particularly insensitive doctor, who announced that I had macular degeneration and "should prepare to cope over time with failing vision." Fifteen minutes later, he was on to the next patient after asking to see me again in a year to monitor my "progress." Furious, I wondered, Progress toward what?

I never saw that doctor again, but I did consult others. Many were more generous with their time and more sensitive in delivering their diagnosis. They also were responsive to my increasingly well-informed questions, many of which were based on data I had gathered for this book.

For eighteen months I read everything I could find on the subject of macular degeneration—from scientific papers presented at symposiums to heartfelt testimonials to the carefully couched promises from vendors of products and therapies outside medical science. I believed that if I knew everything, tried anything, and viewed it all from a logical perspective, then by the time we finished writing the book, I would have all the answers. Well, I don't have all the answers. And I don't have all the sight I want, nor even the sight I had when I began this project. In fact, during months of drafting and retyping, I had to increase the font size on my laptop three times. What I do have now, and hope to pass on to other readers, is a clear understanding of the work being done by medical science to treat the disease, and a comprehensive knowledge of treatment alternatives that have been helpful to other patients.

Macular Degeneration does not sugarcoat the truth. You will learn enough about the medical science of ARMD to feel more comfortable discussing your condition with your eye doctor and more able to ask the right questions before choosing treatments, whether medical or alternative (that is, outside the realm of conventional medical science). You will also hear how other people are coping with ARMD, from how they manage personally and professionally, despite vision problems, to how they felt when undergoing various diagnostic and treatment procedures.

It's important to recognize and attend to the emotional toll macular degeneration takes on your life. ARMD is an *eye* disease. Physically, it does not spread like poison ivy, but it can take over if you let it. That can easily happen, because with ARMD and diminished sight come the potential for a major loss of self-esteem and self-confidence. And this can be a far more debilitating condition than poor vision.

While working on this book, I had surgery on my leg to repair the damage from a serious running accident. On crutches for months, I was forever struggling with heavy doors in public buildings, with hoisting packages into the car, and with finding a seat in a darkened theater. People frequently ran across parking lots to help me; they stopped what they were doing and generously offered to carry packages or to assist me in negotiating curbs. In truth, I had become so accustomed to crutches, and so adept at backpacking even a week's worth of groceries, that I rarely needed much help. At least not because of my leg.

What people perceived as a physical problem was a normal function of my limited sight. I couldn't find the door handle, or I couldn't see the curb, or I couldn't adjust to bright daylight after emerging from a dimly lit restaurant. My hesitancy had nothing to do with my crutches.

After the cast was removed and I had learned to walk again, my sight problems remained, but there were no Boy Scouts leaping to my assistance, no doors being opened for me, no friendly hands offered to guide me. I momentarily longed for another cast, some visible and immediately recognizable symbol of impairment. This experience made me realize that my eye problems had spread to my head and my heart, that gradually I had let myself be transformed into someone with less confidence in my ability to negotiate curbs, both real and metaphorical.

I continue to fight the battle to nurture independence, optimism, and self-confidence. Some days I am triumphant; other days I am less successful. But I am convinced that my eyesight will improve not solely by finding the right doctor or treatment but by maintaining my belief in myself. I am not my disease, but neither are my eyes a segregated body part that can be treated the way I treat a broken pipe in my home. Healing, for me, has meant embracing a range of therapies and techniques, some of which are considered "alternative." Together they improve how I feel, and therefore, I believe, how well I see. This is a very long way from where I started in searching for "the" cure, but it is an approach that has worked for me. I hope this book enables others to find their own personal combination of curative strategies and that they will be able to contemplate a future with clearer sight.

AUTHOR'S NOTE

The use of first-person singular in the text reflects narration by Dr. Robert D'Amato. References to Joan Snyder are clearly identified.

Patients' names and identifying circumstances have been changed to protect the privacy of those whose stories appear in this book.

PART ONE

Understanding and Diagnosing Age-Related Macular Degeneration

1

The Miracle of Eyesight

Macular degeneration is an eye disease that has been described, most recently by ABC's *20/20* TV program, as perhaps *the* most significant epidemic of the twentieth century, affecting 13 million Americans and millions more around the globe. The probability of being afflicted by macular degeneration increases with age, but this is not to say that younger people are not stricken. While the disease can result in a loss of one's central vision, the rate of loss differs widely.

There are several forms of macular degeneration, but the most prevalent is age-related macular degeneration (ARMD), the subject of this book. Despite the name, ARMD can occur at a relatively early age. Arthur Schmidt, for example, is an attorney who was diagnosed with ARMD at the age of fifty-seven.

Arthur first experienced "eye problems" decades ago in law school. He had trouble making out some of the words in his textbooks and often got headaches as he read. He reasoned, quite logically, that eyestrain and fatigue were the cause of his problems. At the student union he was referred to an optician. As soon as he got his first pair of reading glasses, his ability to read without difficulty was instantly restored, and his headaches vanished. Every few years, when the edges of letters grew fuzzy and the lines harder to read, he would visit the optician nearest his law office and get a slightly stronger prescription.

Arthur had learned, without thinking about it, that if reading became more difficult, the proven solution was simply a new pair of spectacles with a stronger correction. He bemoaned the fact that his advancing years were requiring prescription changes ever more frequently, but he didn't give the matter any more thought. Whenever necessary, he visited the optician for a quick fix.

Eventually, he realized that although he could read reasonably well with a brand-new pair of glasses, he could not read perfectly. It took him longer and longer to finish the materials necessary to prepare cases for his clients. Finally, when reading became just too difficult to ignore the problem any longer, Arthur took time out of his busy schedule to consult a good ophthalmologist, a medical doctor who specializes in diseases of the eye.

Arthur Schmidt never suspected he had an eye disease. When his doctor gave him the diagnosis of macular degeneration, Arthur had no idea what a macula was and didn't know he even had one. (In fact, we have two maculae, one in each eye, at the center of the retina.) He had never spent even twenty seconds thinking about the health of his eyes. Like so many people, he took for granted that he had perfectly healthy eyes and that any vision problems could be corrected with glasses.

Arthur's case is far from unusual. Macular degeneration is not a disease that is accompanied by fiercely debilitating symptoms at its onset. There is no eye pain—ever. Isolated as a discrete event, failure to read well, even with properly prescribed glasses, is an obvious sign of some difficulty that should be investigated. But Arthur assumed that as a healthy, middle-aged man, he could expect his vision to "slip a bit each year," as he put it, "just as my hairline did." He paid very little attention to *what* he failed to see when he tried to read, or *how* the lines appeared when he studied them carefully.

THE ANATOMY OF THE EYE

The eye is a remarkable organ. That is the plain and simple truth. When you think of trying to accomplish the ordinary things you do each day without eyesight, you realize immediately how much you depend on your vision. Despite its small size, the eye is one of the most complex organs in the human body, infinitely more complex than even the most sophisticated computer. To understand how macular degeneration and other eye conditions affect eyesight, you need to know how the eye works.

I have been studying human eyes for years, but recently I've been astonished at how quickly we are increasing our understanding of the highly specialized role played by each component of the eye. A thorough knowledge of each component—both its structure and

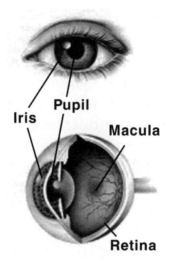

Major parts of the eye.
(Macular Degeneration Foundation)

its function—provides us with clues for solving complex eye problems. This understanding is what enables medical science to make strides toward finding cures for eye diseases such as age-related macular degeneration (ARMD).*

The Front of the Eye

The front, or anterior section, of the eye is composed of the cornea, the pupil, the iris, and the lens.

The cornea is a transparent membrane sitting on the very outside of the eyeball. A resilient substance com-

---

*Age-related macular degeneration is also abbreviated as AMD and MD. The latter is not recommended because it is not precise enough (given that there are several forms of macular degeneration). In some literature, the name senile macular degeneration appears, though it is generally considered outdated and inappropriate.

paratively resistant to damage, the cornea is what is touched when you're accidentally poked in the eye. It is also what gets scratched when a particle lodges between it and a contact lens, creating a very painful but a generally quick-healing injury. The clear cornea is continuous with the white sclera that forms the rest of the outer layer of the eye. An additional thin membrane of clear skin known as the conjunctiva covers all of the eyeball except the cornea.

The pupil, the opening at the center of the colored iris, limits the total brightness of incoming light that is focused by the lens behind it, onto the retina itself.

The Back of the Eye

The back, or posterior section, of the eye is composed of three layers of material. The outermost is the sclera, the membrane that maintains the basic shape of the eye. The second layer of the eye, sandwiched in the middle, is known as the choroid. It is a very thin layer comprising mostly blood vessels. The last and innermost layer is the retina, which contains all the nerve cells that communicate with the optic nerve. The retina is, in effect, the brain's telephone line.

A hardworking tissue, the retina actually uses more oxygen and nutrients per gram of tissue than almost any other part of the body. In order to secure the rapid flow of oxygen and nutrients it requires, the retina is held between two layers of blood vessels. One is a dense carpet of vessels supplying the neurons that process signals for the brain. The other is within the layer known as the choroid. These latter blood vessels supply oxygen to the retinal pigment epithelial cells (RPE cells) and to the light-sensing cells in the retina known as photoreceptors. The RPE and choroid are critical support tissues for the retina. The RPE is a thin layer of cells just under the photoreceptors that helps remove waste products from the retina, maintaining the health of the photoreceptors. The choroid also helps remove retinal waste and brings new supplies of nutrients and oxygen to the retina.

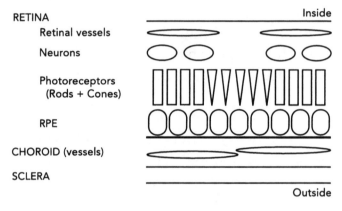

As the figure on page 6 demonstrates, the retina takes up a good deal of the surface behind the eye, but the brain is really most attentive to only a small part of the data the retina sends to it. The macula, an area the size of a pinhead, is in the very center of the retina and is responsible for providing central focus.

The macula enables you, for example, to see the football that is passed on the field, even from bleacher seats. While you watch the ball, you simultaneously see an illegal block downfield, but that event is being processed in the 97 percent of the retina that receives images in the periphery of your vision. The macula, although it represents only 3 percent of the retina, is its most essential component, because it is that tiny sliver that enables us to analyze fine detail.

Certainly no part of the human eye is dispensable, but the orchestrated action of the many separate components within the eye is really the miracle of sight itself. Still, if one part can be said to be functionally harder working than other parts, it would surely be the retina with its multiple layers of vessels, neurons, and photoreceptors, all continuously active.

The photoreceptor layer of the retina contains two types of cells, known as the rods and the cones. The rods are called into action for dim or dark situations. They account for your being able to see a black cat on a starless night, crossing a wooded field. The cones function in bright light or simple daylight. Cone cells also determine your ability to distinguish fine detail and to differentiate color. They account for your being able to see that same cat the next morning on your neighbor's porch, wearing a red and gray collar. The color-sensing cones are concentrated in the macula, and they aid in defining the sharpness of central vision. Rods and cones send their information to another group of cells, the bipolar neuronal cells, which in turn relay the data to ganglion neuronal cells. This is the last transmittal terminal on the way to the brain itself.

The heart of our ability to fixate or focus on one object directly, the cat's pink nose, for example, is lodged in the fovea, a tiny group of cone cells at the very center of the macula. The fovea provides you an unobstructed view of the world directly ahead. In fact, all the blood vessels in front of it are pulled to the sides, like a stage curtain, to create crystal-clear vision. Trouble in the area of the fovea spells trouble in central vision and often in color differentiation. These symptoms frequently lead to a diagnosis of macular degeneration.

HOW WE SEE

Light from a distant object first hits the surface of the cornea, the clear part of the eye, on its outermost surface. Light travels through the cornea and is bent, the first step in the process of focusing the image. The light then travels across a fluid-filled area called the anterior chamber located in front of the lens. Next the light reaches the pupil and lens of the eye. The pupil serves as an aperture that adjusts the overall brightness of the incoming image. The light passing through the pupil is then further bent as it passes through the lens. The lens, unlike the cornea, has the ability to vary the degree to which it bends the light. This is what gives the eye the ability to focus on objects that are at different distances. The closer an object is to the eye, the more the lens must bend the incoming light to keep it in focus on the retina. The rays leaving the lens then travel across a second fluid-filled chamber in the back of the eye known as the vitreous. At this point, the image is ready to be received by the retina, the thin layer of neuronal tissue responsible for interpreting the focused image.

The incoming image is actually flipped upside down as it traverses the lens, but the retina and the brain are able to restore the proper orientation as they process the signal. There are three different layers of cells stacked one upon the other in the retina. Surprisingly, the layer of photoreceptors that detects the light and converts it into electrical impulses is at the bottom of the stack. Thus light must travel through two layers of secondary processing neurons before reaching the light-detecting cells at the bottom of the retina. Photoreceptor cells convert light to electrical signals, which then leave the photoreceptors and backtrack through each of the other two retinal layers where the signal is processed and further sharpened to prepare for transmission to the brain.

The eye functions much like a camera. Light entering through the cornea and through the lens is focused the same way that a camera lens focuses the "picture" of what's in front of it. The focused light or image is projected onto the retina, just as a "picture" is projected onto the film in a camera. The image captured by the retina is then sent to the brain through the optic nerve. This camera-like action is so swift in ordinary light, and normally so reliable, that we take for granted the very sophisticated mechanism that allows it to occur.

In effect, the brain is the commentator for the eye's slide show, and the interpreter of the images that are received. A comprehensive understanding of the pictorial data is essential to vision, because without the brain's interpretive work on the photographic information, we would technically "see" but lack any understanding of what we're seeing. It would be like looking at the various shapes drawn on a sheet of paper without realizing they were the blueprints for a building.

The delicacy of the eye and its many parts are both the reason for its miraculous functioning and the explanation for some of the sight problems that can develop, especially later in life. A machine with millions of parts is expected, periodically, to require some repairs; its very complexity compounds the chances that problems will occur with decades of constant use.

2

⁓

Risk Factors for ARMD

It's impossible to know who will get ARMD. There are approximately 13 million people in the United States alone who are categorized as having this condition. From what we know about the people who have been diagnosed, we can conclude that they have certain traits in common. That doesn't prove that these traits cause ARMD or predict susceptibility, but they do provide indicators that help explain who is more likely to develop ARMD.

DEMOGRAPHICS OF ARMD

Age Groups

By far the most significant correlate for macular disease is age. In one of the most comprehensive studies done to date, researchers found that individuals over seventy-five years of age are roughly six times as likely to develop macular disease as those between the ages of forty-three and fifty-four.* But ARMD begins to be statistically evident in the latter age group, with an incidence of just under 5 percent in the population studied.

According to the same study, more cases are detected in individuals between the ages of fifty-five and sixty-four, but the incidence is still just above 5 percent. Macular degeneration roughly triples, however, in the next age group; for those between the ages of sixty-five and seventy-four, researchers discovered a disease rate of approximately 16 percent.

Two other studies showed somewhat lower rates of detection, but the trend in correlating greater age with greater risk of disease was every bit as evident.

Sex

The Beaver Dam study found that in the age group from forty to sixty, the incidence of age-related macular degeneration is higher among males. But this tendency reverses itself in later years, with more women than men affected in the age group from sixty-five to seventy-four. Among those older than seventy-five, women are almost twice as likely to have ARMD. The reasons for this reversal are not at all clear, though one working hypothesis is that the protective effect of estrogen is lost in postmenopausal women.

Racial Groups

The available data on this parameter are both limited and vaguely contradictory. Blacks and Caucasians have

*The Beaver Dam Eye Study, conducted in Beaver Dam, Wisconsin, in 1988–90, involved 5,924 persons between the ages of forty-three and eighty-six.

Is There an Explanation for ARMD's Epidemic?

There has been a great deal of coverage lately in the print and broadcast media about age-related macular degeneration. It is discussed as a silent thief, robbing elders of their enjoyment of life. But the truth is that ARMD is not all that new. Retinal deterioration, in general, is not uncommon. Nor is macular degeneration the only disease of the retina.

The medical community has been studying the actual phenomenon of macular degeneration for many years, but the fact that many more people are living longer is the real explanation for widespread awareness of the disease now. It is highly probable that had our lifespan not increased so dramatically in the last forty years, there would not have been a corresponding increase in the incidence of the disease itself.

similar rates of early symptom development seen in early ARMD. However, some studies, specifically one that compared English white patients in London with South African black patients, and another in Barbados, have suggested that blacks are far less prone to the later, more severe forms of ARMD than are Caucasians. It is theorized that melanin—the substance that protects the skin from burning, and which is more abundant in blacks than in whites—may protect the eyes. Data on the incidence of ARMD in Hispanics and Asians are extremely scarce, but one study, based on a small sample in Colorado, suggests that ARMD is significantly less frequent among Hispanics than non-Hispanics. It would be useful to have more data and more precisely controlled studies, because often the age groups being compared are different, or other important variables are introduced. These differences make inference easy, but conclusive proof much more difficult.

Family Groups

Like many diseases that researchers are now beginning to understand more clearly, age-related macular degeneration seems to be very closely linked to hereditary factors. If your siblings, parents, or grandparents were afflicted by this condition, there is a greater chance that you will be too. The statistical probabilities are not available, but the correlation may be quite high. A study being conducted at the Massachusetts Eye and Ear Infirmary in Boston, jointly sponsored by the National Institutes of Health and the National Eye Institute, is directed at evaluating families in which there are multiple instances of ARMD.

GENETIC PREDISPOSITION TO ARMD

Regardless of your family history with age-related macular degeneration, there are certain genetic traits that are closely linked to the disease.

Iris Color

People with light-colored eyes (light irides) appear to be at somewhat higher risk of developing ARMD than those with dark irides. The increased risk is thought to be related to lower levels of protective melanin in the eye. It is not quite so simple, though, as thinking that blue- or green-eyed people have more to worry about than those with brown eyes. Eye color often changes during one's lifetime, and the studies on eye color and age-related macular degeneration have not been detailed enough to fully account for this variable.

Farsightedness

The research up to his point does indicate some correlation between being extremely farsighted (i.e., "hyperopic") and the development of both early-stage (dry) and late-stage (wet) ARMD. While we don't yet know the extent of the correlation, or whether being farsighted early in life is a determining factor, available information now suggests that those who see best when objects are far away may be at a slightly higher risk. Hyperopic eyes have not grown fully and are actually shorter than normal eyes when measured from front to back. This slight variation may result in changes in the choroidal vasculature, the maze of blood vessels in the eyes, creating a predisposition to the growth of abnormal blood vessels later in life.

LIFESTYLE AND
ENVIRONMENTAL FACTORS

There is precious little we can do about our family history or our genetic makeup, but there is no question that lifestyle factors that are destructive of good health, especially the health of your eyes, can and should be modified.

Smoking

The data are limited, and the exact causal links fuzzy, but smokers do have a higher rate of age-related macular degeneration than nonsmokers. Even twenty years ago, it was evident from a study conducted by M. E. Paetkau that the onset of ARMD occurred earlier among smokers than nonsmokers.* In another study, involving 1,000 patients, there was a significant correlation between wet ARMD and smoking. Two additional studies, in which nurses and doctors were the subjects, led researchers to estimate that women who smoked twenty-five or more cigarettes per day were more than twice as likely to develop wet ARMD, and the likelihood among male physicians was even higher.† Smokers are also prone to other health problems, such as cardiovascular disease, that can exacerbate vision problems. Of the many ARMD risk factors that are within the control of the individual, the decision to stop smoking is surely the most important.

Sunlight Exposure

If your recreational activities or your occupation exposes you to intense bright sunlight for prolonged periods, you have a greater chance of developing some

*M. E. Paetkau et al., "Senile Disciform Macular Degeneration and Smoking," *Canadian Journal of Ophthalmology* 13:67–71, (1978).
†J. M. Seddon et al., "A Prospective Study of Cigarette Smoking and Age-Related Macular Degeneration in Women," *JAMA* 276:1141–1146 (1996), and W. G. Christen et al., "A Prospective Study of Cigarette Smoking and Risk of Age-Related Macular Degeneration in Men," *JAMA* 276:1147–1151 (1996).

retinal damage late in life. This is not to say that you will necessarily experience any vision loss or even notice any symptoms. However, in some studies bright light exposure has been identified as a risk factor for ARMD.

Supporting this conclusion is the observation that patients with dark irises are less prone to develop ARMD, and dark irises, by definition, limit the incoming light. If bright light exposure (or more probably blue light exposure, the more damaging part of the light spectrum) is linked to the disease, it appears that the problem does not surface until an individual is quite elderly, generally over eighty-five.

We cannot say precisely what impact environmental changes have had on eye health, nor do we know how they will affect eye health in the future. We do know that sunlight is more damaging in some parts of the world than ever before, especially in locations such as Patagonia where holes in the ozone layer have been found. Tracing the effect of these changes over time is a monumental task, and tracking them directly as they impact vision is all but impossible at the moment. There is speculation, however, that climatic and environmental changes have caused an increased incidence of retinal deterioration, both in animals and in humans.

Hypertension

Also known as high blood pressure, hypertension is on the rise in the United States. It may cause damage to retinal vessels and result in retinal bleeding. Atherosclerotic plaques can fragment and obstruct retinal vessels, producing a form of stroke in the eye. At least one major analysis of patients with ARMD found a prevalence of high blood pressure among the study group. The condition also worsened more quickly among those with higher blood pressure. A recent study by L. Hyman and associates showed that there was significant association of diastolic blood pressure (the numerator of the statistic) over 95 mm Hg and wet ARMD.*

Although people can do nothing about the color of their eyes, their grandmother's age-related macular degeneration, or the fact that they need reading glasses, they can be aware that they, perhaps to a greater degree than others, need to be more mindful of changes in their vision and more diligent about going for a thorough medical checkup of their eyes. Collecting data on the common characteristics of ARMD patients is also crucial to medical researchers. Evaluating such data leads them to an ever-clearer understanding of the possible causes of ARMD, which facilitates work toward a cure.

*L. Hyman et al., "Risk Factors for Age-Related Maculopathy," *Investigative Ophthalmology and Visual Science,* 33:801 (1992).

3

Recognizing and Understanding ARMD

All of us can see better on some days than on others. This is as true for people with nearly perfect vision as it is for people with poor eyesight. Factors such as fatigue, stress, or allergies can have a temporary impact on our ability to see clearly. Adelle Ross, one of the patients in my clinic, tells me that her favorite weekend ritual is sitting at the kitchen table with a steaming cup of hot coffee, leisurely leafing through the newspaper and enjoying the luxury of unscheduled time. She gazes through the large kitchen windows onto the New England village street where she lives, and revels in the changing landscape as the seasons come and go. But when spring arrives with its first crocuses, she also notices that some of the details of the street life are occasionally less distinct. The picket fence across the yard is a bit blurry, and tears make even her newspaper difficult to read.

Adelle's experience is very common, and she knows

that there is no reason to assume she is developing a serious eye disease. Spring flowers bring on seasonal allergies, and transient blurry eyesight is often a temporary, self-correcting consequence. But if you sit at your kitchen table sipping coffee every morning, and if over a period of time the street sign and other familiar landmarks become less distinct, you need to find out why. To do so, you should consult a professional eye doctor.

VISION SPECIALISTS

There are three types of vision specialists: opticians, optometrists, and ophthalmologists.

Opticians are technicians qualified to grind lenses to the precise specifications of your current eye prescription, and to fit you properly with eyeglasses or contact lenses. They are well versed in the myriad corrective options available to consumers, who may be trying to decide, for example, between bifocals and progressive lenses, or between antireflective coatings and tinted lenses. Their experience is as crucial in selecting a pair of comfortable glasses for the individual as the optometrist's is in prescribing the best correction for the lenses.

An *optometrist* is an individual with a minimum of four years of training in optometry school and generally four or more years of college studies. This professional is also known as a doctor of optometry—hence the initials *O.D.* following his or her name—and, in a few states, as an optometric physician. An optometrist is allowed to prescribe some ophthalmic medications but does not perform surgery. The science of optometry concerns itself with the range and the power of vision.

Where the range or power is inadequate, the optometrist can in most cases prescribe the amount of refraction, or correction, to give the patient 20/20 vision. Most optometrists also fit and sell the contact lenses or glasses their patients require, but if your optometrist does not, you will need to visit an optician.

An *ophthalmologist* is a medical doctor who has completed four years of college, four years of medical school, one year of internship, and three years of residency in a hospital. In this book, the term *eye doctor* will be used to refer to an ophthalmologist. These physicians are highly trained in diseases of the eye. Many complete an additional two-year fellowship to specialize in retinal disorders (such as ARMD), surgical retinal disorders (such as retinal detachments), glaucoma, corneal problems, pediatrics, or plastic surgery. Glaucoma, cataracts, and other eye problems, though not necessarily the direct result of aging, are all more common in older people. If you are over fifty-five, you should visit an ophthalmologist once a year.

Within each of these three professions, there are specialists who work exclusively or primarily with low-vision patients, meaning those who have uncorrectable vision problems. Some states, such as New York, have a qualifying certification procedure for low-vision optometrists; others, such as California, do not. If your state *does* have credential verification (a fact you can check through your local congressional representative's office), and particularly if you have been diagnosed with ARMD, you should certainly consult a specialist who has been certified. Because of their training and experience in the field, low-vision specialists have great

familiarity with the particular problems of their patients, and they can recommend the visual aids that are
most helpful to them. Thus it is generally more appropriate for most ARMD patients to see such specialists
rather than generalists.

SYMPTOMS

Most people over fifty benefit from a complete baseline
eye examination by an ophthalmologist whether they
sense any change in their vision or not. Early detection
is essential for optimal results in the treatment of virtually any disease, and conditions of the eyes are no exception. You are your own best eye doctor in the sense
that you will notice, if you are attentive, the important
changes in your sight. It is the ophthalmologist's job to
then diagnose the cause of your vision problems and
work toward the cure or correction, which may be as
simple as a new pair of glasses.

As a specialized medical research doctor in the field
of ophthalmology, I am often consulted by people who
have noticed their vision "slipping" and have gone to
the optometrist for their first pair of glasses or, if they
already wear glasses, for a stronger prescription. Very
frequently, they conclude that their vision improved
with the new glasses, but only temporarily. People have
also come to me complaining that their eyesight is deteriorating at a faster rate as they're growing older. They
often say that after repeated expenditures for new
glasses, each pair stronger than the last, they still can't
achieve the visual acuity that they had earlier.

Vision is primarily subjective. There is no reliable

way to measure eyesight other than by one's own responses to the same question posed over and over as different corrective lenses are held in front of each eye. "Is it better this way, or that way?" "Clearer here, or here?" As the "choices" all begin to look alike, the question of preference begins to seem unanswerable. One correction may in fact enable you to see *better* than another lens, but it does not guarantee that you will see *perfectly*. Concentrating carefully and telling your doctor which corrective lens gives you the sharper vision does not necessarily ensure that you will leave with a prescription that gives you 20/20 vision.

This dilemma is often the experience of people ultimately diagnosed with macular degeneration, because in its early stages there may be only subtle changes in their eyesight, none of which may be dramatic enough to suggest disease. Many of us are not especially mindful of minor changes in our vision because perfect acuity isn't always required. Often it is only in a comparative context, when we look at the same faces on the train each morning or pass the same billboard, that we begin to notice diminished acuity or even more peculiar symptoms.

Common symptoms among patients diagnosed with age-related macular degeneration include the following:

- When reading, even with corrective lenses, letters or lines appear distorted.
- There may be a fuzzy, blurry spot or pieces may be "missing" when you stare directly at one word or one letter.
- Road signs or even highway signs with very large letters are difficult to read.

- There is a dark spot or a "blank" spot in the center of your vision. When you look at a red stoplight, the red part may seem to disappear, but you have no difficulty noticing when the green light comes on.
- Straight edges, like those of doorways or windowsills, look wavy or crooked.
- Color vision is less acute; colors of towels or clothing that you remember being very bright may seem dull or even another shade.
- It's difficult to see well in the dark, or when lighting is low, you have trouble making out the edge of the stairs or sidewalks.

These symptoms suggest that there may be a problem with the macula. This area, where central vision is processed, differs from the rest of the retina so that changes in the macula do not affect peripheral, or side, vision. Macular degeneration is basically experienced as the deterioration of straightforward vision, whereby looking directly at someone and meeting that person's eyes becomes virtually impossible.

Different types of macular degeneration can cause slightly different symptoms, and in the beginning stages, it is not always easy to describe the exact nature of the vision difficulty. Because a "good" eye will compensate for a "weak" eye, the sight you have on average may be so little changed that you can barely detect any difficulty. You may just have the sense that your vision is slightly less acute sometimes, especially if you operate in a familiar environment and don't need to see perfectly to perform routine tasks. Or you may think you need stronger lighting in your home because hazy vision is often interpreted merely as insufficient illumination, especially for close work such as sewing or reading. And indeed, brighter light may help somewhat; but if macular degeneration is the problem, brighter lights are not really a solution.

One of the most confusing characteristics of macular degeneration is that peripheral vision is unimpaired. Patients will frequently make remarks to me like the following: "I have difficulty focusing when I read the newspaper, but I'm not sure there's anything wrong with my eyesight, because I can see the cat dart in and out between planter boxes, even from the corner of my eye." Why is it that you have trouble reading but are perfectly able to see images on the periphery, even fleeting ones?

The explanation for this seeming paradox is that the retina has essentially two distinct functions: One provides for direct, central vision, the other for peripheral vision. It is the macula that enables you to see straight ahead and to perform tasks such as knitting or fly-tying; the remainder of the retina, more than 90 percent of it, is designed to provide images that are on the edges, or periphery, of your field of vision. If the macula is deteriorating, only your central vision will be impaired. Everything you see to the side will be crystal clear and totally unaffected.

SCREENING

If you suspect you have ARMD, you need to go for a complete eye examination. In a routine exam the doctor will not only evaluate your vision but also check the health of your eyes. Looking at each eye with a slit lamp or a high-powered microscope, the doctor determines if the corneas are clear (free of scarring or infection) and if cataracts are forming on the lenses (which might cloud your vision). Then the pressure in your eyes is evaluated to test for glaucoma; at this point, eye drops are administered to assist the doctor in looking at your retinas.

The drops cause each pupil to enlarge, giving the ophthalmologist a better view of the retina on the back inside wall of the eye. (See the diagram of the eye in chapter 1.) Typically, the doctor will examine the retina with an indirect ophthalmoscope. This device, which is attached to a helmetlike structure worn on the ophthalmologist's head, has a magnifying lens and a light that facilitate detailed viewing of the retina. This step in the examination can be unpleasant for some patients because the light is very bright, uncomfortably so for anyone with light sensitivity. More than one patient has told me it is the exact sensation remembered from childhood play when an older sibling held you down with your eyelids forced open, and shined a flashlight directly into your eyes. But in the doctor's office, the examination is relatively brief and absolutely essential.

Often the ophthalmologist will place a special lens over the patient's eye to magnify the retina. A perfectly clear retina will look pink or rosy. The macula will appear as a round, orange spot in the middle of the retina. In the very center of the macula the doctor will see the fovea, the part of the macula responsible for the sharpest vision. It is the human eye's "spyglass," which enables us to spot small objects far away—a fox across a field, a ship far out to sea.

The first sign of macular degeneration visible to an

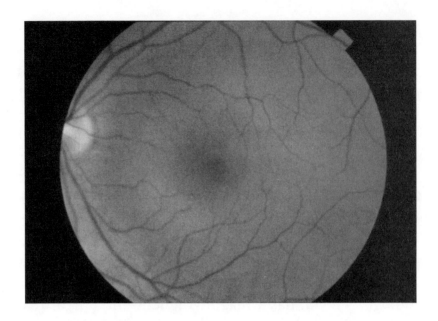

A healthy retina (*above*) *(National Eye Institute, National Institutes of Health)* and a retina with drusen typical of dry ARMD (*below*). *(The New York Ear & Eye Infirmary)*

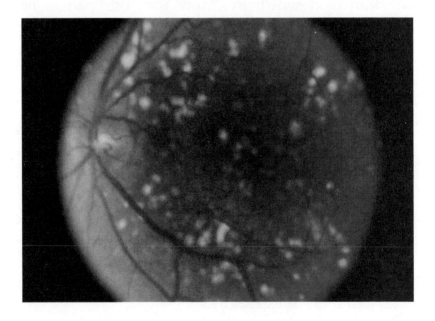

ophthalmologist is the appearance of *drusen,* or little yellow dots under the retina. There may be only a few dots, or there may be many; the number is not necessarily consistent with the degree of vision impairment. In fact, drusen may be present in a patient who has no symptoms of eye disease whatsoever, one who may not even wear glasses. There are many people over the age of fifty-five, some even younger, who, in routine eye examinations, discovered that they had a substantial number of drusen. But they had experienced no symptoms of disease and certainly had no sense of failing vision. During a routine eye exam, you should ask your own ophthalmologist if there are any drusen evident on the retina of either eye. If there are, you need to be especially attentive to any changes in your vision that may occur in the future.

Medical science does not know the significance of drusen, nor what role they may have in predicting vision problems. Current scientific thought suggests that drusen represent the buildup of waste material from cells, which in a perfectly healthy eye would be removed naturally by the body. Just as your morning shower washes away dead cells from your skin, blood flow in a healthy eye washes away waste from photoreceptor cells in the retina. But this process functions abnormally when the eye is diseased with macular degeneration; therefore drusen build up in the retina.

It is not clear that the drusen themselves are particularly troublesome or even cause vision loss. We do know, however, that these little yellow dots can be the precursors of a more serious development: the growth of new blood vessels in the eye. When new blood vessels grow under drusen, they tend to leak fluid, which causes a distortion of the overlying retina and subsequent vision loss. Such growth, however, is *not* inevitable when drusen are present; only 10 to 15 percent of the drusen-affected population later develops new blood vessels. Perhaps if we all lived to be 150 years old, everyone with drusen eventually *would* develop abnormal blood vessels in the eyes. But at the moment, we know very little about the timing of or the reasons for what we assume to be this "second stage" of macular degeneration.

In the view of many ophthalmologists, the presence of drusen alone warrants a diagnosis of "dry" macular degeneration, even if there is no loss of vision. But when blood vessels appear under the retina, the diagnosis changes to the more troublesome "wet" macular degeneration. It is the wet form of macular degeneration that is almost always associated with serious loss of central vision. Some patients with drusen may also experience difficulty with direct vision; others may not. Researchers are currently trying to determine if drusen actually *cause* new blood vessels to grow, forcing the retina to rise up like a sidewalk where tree roots have lifted the cement, or if these drusen are merely a sign of an initial degenerative process that may later progress to the wet stage. If they can determine that the drusen are causal, medical researchers can focus on prevention of drusen or some methodology that would enhance the eye's natural ability to carry away cellular waste. If drusen are merely associated with an event that 90 percent of the affected population won't experience, research efforts can be focused on effective treatments of the blood vessels themselves and, better yet, a way to prevent their development.

If your ophthalmologist does indeed see drusen under your retina, and if you have expressed concerns about your vision changing, he or she may refer you to a retinal specialist. Whether you get a referral or not, it is wise to consult such a specialist, who deals with macular deterioration on a daily basis and thus has more experience in diagnosing and treating the condition. (Later in this chapter, we'll take a closer look at drusen and the various forms of ARMD.)

Sandra Robbins's story illustrates the insidious way in which age-related macular degeneration can alter one's vision, and the consequences that may result when one is inattentive to or ignores even subtle changes in vision.

Sandra is an accomplished painter. For twenty years she has created idyllic seascapes reflecting the beauty of the California shoreline where she lives. With the experience of many canvases behind her, Sandra knows her palette well, mixing the same shades over and over for use in ever more highly stylized presentations. Periodically she would conclude that her palette had become dull, but then dismissed the idea as excessive self-criticism.

One morning she set about filling in color on a seascape already sketched out by her assistant, and found, much to her surprise, that her customary colors all looked more muted than usual. The next morning, the sensation was even more acute. What had been her signature color palette had suddenly faded to something that looked, to her, like nothing more than muted tones of gray. Worse yet, lines that she knew she had painted as straight suddenly looked wavy and distorted.

Sandra had no eye doctor, having never experienced even the need for reading glasses. Through friends she was referred to an ophthalmologist, who, after examining her eyes, suggested she see a retinal specialist. There she was told that wet macular degeneration had apparently compromised one eye some time ago, though Sandra had no idea that she had become highly dependent on the *other* eye. When suddenly the "good" eye developed the same problems, her compromised color perception seemed like an overnight phenomenon. In fact, it was much longer in coming but wasn't apparent—not even to a woman whose profession depended heavily upon her eyesight.

Macular degeneration has not ended Sandra's career as a painter. Where she used to pick up stark contrasts in colors, she now sees subtle differences, but her artistry is undiminished.

Since progression of the disease is unpredictable— fast in some patients, all but imperceptible over decades in others—it is essential that you monitor your condition closely if you've been diagnosed with age-related macular degeneration. At the moment, ARMD cannot be reversed, but clinical trials are under way that may enable us to arrest it or slow its progression.

Whether or not you have been diagnosed with ARMD or with another eye disease, it is important to pay close attention to both sudden and progressive changes in your sight. Early detection of any abnormality provides the optimum chance for proper treatment.

UNDERSTANDING WHAT DRUSEN ARE

With specialized magnifiers, an experienced ophthalmologist can recognize drusen instantly. Not all drusen are alike, however; they differ in color, in shape, in number, configuration, and elevation. All these parameters can be measured, some with more accuracy than others, but the most important distinction in characterizing drusen is whether they are hard or soft.

Hard drusen are generally small, round, and flat, though a number of them may be grouped together, suggesting the appearance of one large drusen. According to one expert in the field of macular degeneration, Dr. Maureen G. Maguire, "Hard drusen alone are not considered an indication of early AMD, since they are present in one or both eyes of nearly 100% of the population aged 43 years or older. . . . *their presence and number are not associated with increased risk of the late forms of AMD.*"* (emphasis added) This fact is extremely important to bear in mind if you are informed by your ophthalmologist that you have hard drusen and therefore have macular degeneration.

Consider, for example, the case of Stefie Wexler, a successful interior decorator. She knew a lot about ARMD because her husband, Seth, had this condition. Fortunately for Seth, he was already retired when he was diagnosed, so his ARMD did not interfere with his

*Jeffrey W. Berger, Stuart L. Fine, and Maureen G. Maguire, *Age-Related Macular Degeneration* (St. Louis: Mosby, 1999), chapter 2, "Natural History," p. 17.

career. He was less fortunate in experiencing both rapid and serious deterioration of his eyesight. Shortly after diagnosis, he had a bleeding choroidal blood vessel in the right eye; less than two months later, the same problem developed in the left eye.

Stefie, who was twenty years younger than Seth, had anticipated the possibility of caring for a husband with age-related illnesses, and she actually enjoyed Seth's dependence on her. She helped him coordinate his wardrobe, read the sports page of the newspaper to him, and assisted him in myriad other ways. But when Stefie was told by her ophthalmologist that she was developing drusen in one eye, her world was shattered. She knew, or thought she knew, that it was only a matter of time before she would no longer be able to assist her husband.

For over a year, she remained silent on the subject of her eyesight, which in fact was reasonably good except for a mild correction for reading. Her denial was so complete that she refused to think about returning to her ophthalmologist the next year for her annual exam. But when his office called her to remind her, she faced her fear and forced herself to go for a checkup. This time, she saw a colleague of her regular doctor, who reported, "Yes, I see here a few, insignificant drusen in your left eye that showed up during last year's exam. They look harmless enough, consistent with your early-fifties age group; there's no reason to expect any deterioration, but be sure to let us know if you experience changes in your vision."

Stunned by these remarks, Stefie was a woman reborn. She learned, belatedly, that not all drusen are created equal. Like many people whose only exposure to

ARMD is through the experience of someone whose sight is severely compromised, she had assumed that the word *drusen* is a guarantee of rapid vision loss. Nothing could be further from the truth. It depends on what type of drusen you have. So after hearing the word *drusen* during an ophthalmic examination, you need to find out whether you have hard or soft drusen.

Soft drusen are larger than hard drusen and generally look yellowish gray under the microscope. Whereas hard drusen have distinct borders, soft drusen have indistinct, or fuzzy, edges and resemble a drop of ink on a paper towel. Patients with numerous soft drusen are at higher risk than those with hard drusen for progression to the wet form of ARMD.

Pigmentary abnormalities of the retina are also seen in some patients. Like freckles or age spots on older skin, these variations in what is ordinarily a rosy pink macular pigment may merely suggest that the patient is over fifty. But accumulated data tell us that these variations may also be precursors of macular degeneration. Although not directly related as far as we know, we frequently find excessive pigment clumping in eyes with hard drusen as well as those with soft drusen. Pigment clumping is found sometimes overlying soft drusen too. In the general population, the prevalence of pigmentary abnormality increases with both the size of the largest drusen in the eye as well as with the age of the patient. The bottom line is that the more pigmentary changes and soft drusen you have, the higher your risk of developing the more severe form of ARMD.

While the presence of drusen is not necessarily conclusive evidence of eye disease, the size and type of drusen may be indicative of later developments that will generally be classified as age-related macular degeneration. Unfortunately, we must say "generally categorized" because even an expert panel of doctors assembled from all over the world had differing views on an exact definition of early ARMD.

CLASSIFICATIONS OF ARMD

There are many diseases that affect the macula, some of which (rod/cone dystrophy, for example, or central serous chorioretinopathy) have symptoms very similar to those of ARMD. But these diseases are very different from ARMD in their clinical course, treatment, and outcome. Thus it is critically important for your eye doctor to define with certainty the exact type of macular disease you are dealing with and to explain it to you before you decide on a course of action.

ARMD takes three distinct forms: dry, wet, and pigment epithelial detachment (PED).

Dry ARMD

This form of ARMD is most often described as a collection of clinical signs. These signs include large, soft drusen and pigmentary abnormalities. Rarely are the clinical indicators alone associated with a serious diminution of sight, though the ability to see fine detail may be compromised. Approximately 85 to 90 percent of people with age-related macular degeneration have this dry form, which is less severe, and less debilitating, than the wet form.

On rare occasions, the dry form will progress to a stage called dry "atrophic" macular degeneration, in which the retina becomes thinned in areas with drusen.

While there can be significant loss of vision from atrophic ARMD, the vision loss occurs gradually, in contrast to wet macular degeneration, which most frequently is experienced with more sudden and more significant impairment.

Wet ARMD

Wet ARMD is evidenced most often by choroidal neovascularization, or CNV. This means that new, abnormal blood vessels are growing just under the retina, from the tissue bed known as the choroid. These blood vessels may leak fluid or bleed, lifting up a portion of the overlying retina. Distorted vision almost always results from this leakage, as does serious vision loss. The effect is similar to what happens to a picture in the newspaper when the paper is left out in the rain. Where a lot of moisture has pooled, the surface of the photo looks distorted or even unrecognizable. Ten to 15 percent of ARMD patients will progress from the dry to the wet form of this disease.

If you have wet ARMD, you may hear the term *disciform scar* used to describe the condition of your retina. This scar, so far as medicine can discern right now, is the end result of the CNV process described above. The abnormal blood vessel may have stopped leaking or bleeding, but the results of its leakage are now evident as a type of scar. At this stage it is the scar, not the blood vessel itself, that actually interferes with your sight.

Pigment Epithelial Detachment (PED)

A comparatively rare and distinct form of macular degeneration, PED can and does exist on its own, but more often it is seen in conjunction with CNV. Fluid from the choroid forces the detachment of the overlying retinal pigment epithelial cells away from the membrane to which they are normally attached. PED takes the form of a blister or bump on your retina, and you will likely experience blurred or distorted vision. The fluid causing a PED is typically due to a leaking blood vessel—in other words, a CNV. Sometimes, however, many drusen will consolidate, becoming large enough to be recategorized as a PED. In this type of situation, the large amount of yellow waste material resulting from that consolidated mass of drusen causes detachment of the retinal pigment epithelial cells.

"Early Stage" Versus "Late Stage"

One frequently hears the terms *early stage* and *late stage* in connection with ARMD, suggesting a linear progression that is in fact inconsistent with the disease. There are no clinical divisions of early and late, only clinical definitions of dry and wet. Although it would be highly unusual for someone to walk into an ophthalmologist's office with a serious case of wet ARMD without having experienced some noticeable vision problems over a period of months or years, experiences that would constitute "early-stage" warning signs, no one can logically conclude that "early-stage" dry macular degeneration will automatically progress to some "late stage" of severe atrophy or leaking blood vessels. Do not be alarmed by "stage" vocabulary; it is essentially shorthand for medical professionals, and not a harbinger of any timeline in a disease that may be static for a lifetime.

Classification Scheme for ARMD

No Disease Diagnosis Warranted	*Evidence of Dry (Early-Stage) ARMD*	*Evidence of Wet (Late-Stage) ARMD*
Few hard drusen present	Large, soft drusen, pigment changes	CNV, extensive atrophy, disciform scarring, or PED present

4

~~

The Right Diagnosis

When a doctor informs you that you have a disease, your first reaction is likely to be fear. When the fear subsides enough for you to start thinking clearly again, you probably will think about getting a second medical opinion and having every diagnostic test that could confirm the existence of your condition and establish its severity.

Age-related macular degeneration is not a cooperative disease in this regard. In the first place, even the ARMD diagnosis itself is not clear-cut. Some ophthalmologists believe that the presence of one large druse constitutes proof of the disease. Others believe that many drusen must be present, and that they must be accompanied by visual deterioration.

Even diagnostic tests are not definitive and identify only imprecisely the population of people who should at least statistically be counted as having age-related macular degeneration. The single test that is currently available to us to identify the advanced form of macular degeneration is angiography. Angiography is a tool that pinpoints the precise location of blood vessels that are new and are leaking, vessels that may be candidates for laser treatment.

ANGIOGRAPHY

When your ophthalmologist suspects you may have ARMD after examining your eyes, it is likely that you will be referred for a test known as a fluorescein angiogram. What is the purpose of this test and the value of the data it produces?

Fluorescein angiography gives your doctor additional information about the condition of the interior of your eye by illuminating detail that is not easy to detect, even with sophisticated magnification. Angiography is a branch of diagnostic medicine that deals chiefly with blood vessels. Sodium fluorescein is a substance that emits a green fluorescence when it is exposed to blue light. When doctors began administering fluorescein dye intravenously to examine the vasculature, or the blood vessels, of the retina in the late 1960s, it became evident that this technique could be helpful to patients with macular degeneration, providing useful detailed information about the type and nature of their disease. The procedure itself has changed very little in the last thirty years, but interpretation of the images has evolved into a highly specialized science.

Like so many who hear the message "It looks as though you might have age-related macular degeneration," Burt Freid has only a dim remembrance of the second half of his doctor's sentence: "and I'd like you to get a test to give us more information about your eyes." He knows he left his ophthalmologist's office with a card in his hand indicating the time and date of the next appointment, but he was too anxiety ridden about the initial diagnosis to concentrate on what the next step meant.

"When I did show up for the angiography appointment," Burt recalls, "I didn't know what to expect, how to prepare myself, or whether it was really a treatment or a test. When I finally gathered my wits and started to ask questions, the nurses and technicians were all too busy and too overscheduled to really walk me through the procedure in advance." Ten years later, Burt has been through a number of angiographic tests, which he thinks of no differently from having his teeth cleaned at the dentist or his blood pressure taken by a nurse. But the first was hard because he was both concerned about the diagnosis and uninformed about the test itself.

"I started feeling slightly nauseous when the process began that first time," Burt remembers, "but I understand now that my own anxiety was probably nine-tenths of the problem. I've never felt sick when I've had an angiogram after that first one . . . though I confess that I always now take a can of ginger ale to sip . . . the best advice I can offer is to simply know what's going to happen . . . which, frankly, isn't much."

The process is straightforward. The first picture is a baseline photograph to be used for comparison. A special camera is used to take a rapid sequence of black-and-white photographs of the retina. When a harmless dye is injected into the bloodstream through a vein in your arm, it travels quickly to the retina. Blue light is then used to "excite" the fluorescein dye as it travels through the retinal blood vessels. A highly trained specialist sits before the patient and takes snapshots of the retina over the course of twenty minutes. During this period, the glowing dye tells an interesting story.

Initially, all blood vessels in the retina are lit up by the dye, but it is quickly diluted in the body, except where new blood vessels have grown. In these vessels, the dye remains visible for a longer period of time. A trained observer will see, in the late frames of the test, something like a dust mop or a fuzz ball. This configuration suggests leakage in some of the blood vessels and thus the presence of neovascularization, or "wet" macular degeneration.

Fluorescein angiography is essential for tracking changes in advanced ARMD; in patients with dry ARMD, the procedure can detect patterns of drusen formation that may be precursors to wet ARMD. Not all doctors recommend the test for those with dry ARMD, but even in the case of a healthy patient, it can serve as a baseline against which later tests are compared. A close analogy can be drawn with an electrocardiogram test for healthy patients with a family history of heart disease. Many cardiologists recommend that you take an EKG early in life to establish the baseline data on your normal heartbeat, thus providing comparative grounds for evaluation of even the subtlest changes later in life. Although useful as a baseline, fluorescein angiography is not essential in following dry macular degeneration unless one is suspicious that new blood vessels have begun to grow.

Some patients have obvious drusen as seen through ordinary ophthalmology equipment, but they are asymptomatic and remain without complaint. In my judgment, these patients should have a baseline angiogram if these drusen are large and grouped in a mass, but they don't need another angiogram until symptoms develop or their ophthalmologist detects signs of new blood vessel growth such as the presence of blood or fluid under the retina. In general, fluorescein angiography is a safe procedure. The only adverse reactions reported in a recent study were nausea and itching, and these reactions were found in less than 1 percent of the subjects.*

When an ophthalmologist reviews an angiogram, he or she is usually searching for signs of new blood vessel growth that will damage the retina. The angiogram is also useful for detecting thinning or atrophy of the retina, sometimes seen in severe varieties of dry ARMD. Detailed analysis of new vessel growth can also be of importance in treatment, providing the coordinates for future destruction of the vessel by laser surgery.

A new type of angiography has been introduced that, according to some ophthalmologists, has certain advantages over the use of fluorescein. Known as indocyanine green (ICG) angiography, it uses a water-soluble dye of tricarbocyanine instead of sodium fluorescein. Though the dye acts a bit differently in the body, binding with protein in the blood, it is designed to perform essentially the same function as more traditional angiogra-

*B. J. Jennings and D. E. Mathews, "Adverse Reactions During Retinal Fluorescein Angiography," *Journal of the American Optometric Association* 65, no. 7 (July 1994).

phy. Some ophthalmologists believe the ICG test gives
a brighter signal, allowing a better view of the choroid,
one of the layers just beneath the retina. This is where
new blood vessels grow in wet ARMD.

ANTICIPATING ANGIOGRAPHY

Any test that involves injection of a substance into the
blood can cause anxiety. The very notion of a foreign
substance circulating in the bloodstream is unpleasant,
even if we know the procedure is deemed entirely safe.
Here are some of the most frequently asked questions
put to me by patients:

Q. How is the dye injected?

A. A needle is inserted in a vein, usually in your
arm, and approximately 5 cc's of solution are inserted, an amount roughly equal to a teaspoon.

Q. What will I feel when the dye begins to circulate in my bloodstream?

A. Apart from the unpleasantness of the initial
prick of the needle, there is rarely any awareness at
all that the dye has been released. A small percentage
of patients experience momentary nausea, approxi-

mately sixty to ninety seconds of mild stomach upset, that results from a reaction to the fluorescein.

Q. How is the test conducted?

A. Your eyes will be dilated to offer the widest possible view of the retina. Seated with your forehead against a bar rest, you will be asked to look straight ahead and to refrain from blinking while the technician takes snapshots of your retina, its blood vessels, and the course of the dye over several minutes. It is sometimes difficult to keep one's eyes wide open during all the shots, particularly if you are sensitive to light or light flashes. The technician is trained, however, to anticipate your need to blink periodically and only will ask you for your best efforts. A skilled "filmmaker" will get all the necessary snapshots no matter how many times you blink. Once the initial photos are taken, you will be asked to return in ten minutes for additional photos to identify the staining pattern of new blood vessels.

Q. If I have been diagnosed with ARMD in one eye, will the doctor recommend angiography in *both* eyes?

A. Generally it is wise to check both eyes, even if your complaint is with one eye or if symptoms are revealed in only one eye. Having ARMD in one eye increases your odds of developing it in your other eye; therefore it's important to monitor developments in the good eye as well. Some doctors prefer to administer the test to each eye on different days so that they can get the best photos of one eye rather than alternating between eyes during the test.

Q. Are there any aftereffects of the test?

A. It takes roughly four to six hours for your pupils to return to their normal size after they've been dilated, the same amount of time it would take if you were having your eyes dilated without special attention to ARMD. You will also notice that your urine is slightly orange yellow, a sign that your body is expelling the dye. Drink plenty of water to flush the dye out; it will be gone within twenty-four hours in any event.

Q. Can I look at the films from my angiography and see what the doctor is looking for?

A. There is no reason a doctor would not show you the films, though they are a bit more inscrutable than many medical pictorials. Even ophthalmologists require specialized training to read the results accurately. If you are interested in seeing your films, ask your doctor to review them with you and to point out to you the blood vessels that are particularly troublesome or the drusen that may lead to later problems.

OPTICAL COHERENCE TOMOGRAPHY

OCT is a comparatively new diagnostic tool that offers promise in the management of ARMD. It is an imaging technique, similar to an ultrasound, but it uses light waves to create cross-sectional views of eye tissue. Its greatest value is in the precision of the images it produces, giving ophthalmologists a far more detailed picture of the topography of the retina than would be provided by an angiogram. OCT is not widely available in every part of the United States or the world, but it is an advanced technological tool that can be accessed at many teaching hospitals.

Those who have experienced an OCT diagnostic procedure find that it is far easier and quicker than fluorescein angiography. Besides that, the colorful end product is vastly more interesting to the patient than black-and-white photos produced with an angiogram. According to one patient, "It produces a lovely topographic map of my eye that looks quite like a picture in a geography book." OCT complements but does not *replace* angiography in delineating the presence of new blood vessels.

SELF-SCREENING FOR VISION PROBLEMS

One of the cleverest things our eyes do is deceive us. When one eye is not up to doing its job, the other effectively "compensates." This creative assist is accomplished by the brain, which integrates the signals coming from each eye. When eye problems develop, the compensatory behavior of the stronger eye is both good and bad. It enables you to think you are seeing as well as you always have, but it also marks the development of significant problems.

Pamela Alvarez works as a toll taker on the Massachusetts Turnpike, and during rush hour, she makes change for dozens of drivers every hour. "I had done the job for so long, I thought I could actually see the bill before the driver had taken it from his wallet," she recalls. "I would make the change ready and hand it back in five seconds flat." Speed and accuracy were her daily challenge. "Suddenly, very suddenly, I found I not only couldn't see the amount of the bill when the driver passed it through the window, I could barely make out whether it was a one or a five or a ten, even in the light of the booth.

"My husband suggested that probably my left eye was deteriorating, because drivers always pass on my left. He said, 'Why don't you just get a pair of glasses that has a plain glass in the right eye and magnification in the left. Or better yet, just switch places with someone on the other side of the toll and use your stronger right eye.'

"Brilliant, I thought . . . how simple. I covered what I assumed was my 'weak' left eye and looked at the bill my husband handed me. I was astonished to find that I could see very little at all and might not have even recognized that it was money he was handing me, had I not been told in advance."

Pamela's story is actually not so very unusual. She had no idea that vision in her right eye was so restricted until her left eye had weakened to the point that she was forced to pay attention. Her left eye had, in fact, deteriorated, but it was the right eye that had the more serious deficiency, a deficiency that had been well concealed when her left eye was able to do double duty.

Eye disease always reveals itself to us sooner or later with vision problems. Often, however, it is later rather than sooner. By then, treatment may be somewhat less effective, and progression of disease quite advanced. If you have been diagnosed with age-related macular degeneration, you should ask your ophthalmologist, during every exam, whether there are more drusen evident, or whether any other developments have occurred, even if your vision has not changed since the last exam. If you have not been diagnosed with ARMD but there is a history of it in your family, it is important to remain alert to the possibilities that you may also be at risk for disease. As new treatments and screening procedures become available, you may want to become a participant in clinical trials, and your baseline data could be crucial in measuring the impact of new procedures.

Self-awareness of your own vision is the single most important diagnostic tool for dealing with ARMD. Even the most subtle changes may prove to be significant early warning signs. Keep an "Eye Diary" describing the changes in your vision that concern you. Be aware of sight differences in each eye, covering one, then the other, when looking at specific objects both near and far. Rosa Lane told her doctors that she was seeing new "blips" in her lasered eyes, both of which had exhibited wet ARMD in the past. Although the doctors were skeptical that their patient could actually experience and articulate changes that were not apparent from a retinal exam, Rosa's self-diagnosis was later verified by the angiogram. "You were right," one of her doctors said, pointing out the minuscule amount of new bleeding revealed in the image of Rosa's left eye.

Keep an Amsler Grid (see chapter 6) in your pocket, on your desk, or bookmarked on your Internet browser. Checking the grid daily to assess changes in your vision will give your treating physician the best, most consistent, and accurate data on the status of your eyesight.

5

The Likely Course of ARMD

When you know you have a medical condition, it is natural to want to know what to expect. Being prepared for the probable outcomes, while being open to any possibility, is undoubtedly the best way to cope. Knowledge of future developments, however unwanted those developments may be, can give you a sense of empowerment and calm your fears. But age-related macular degeneration is a disease with a highly unpredictable course of progression: It can progress quickly in some individuals, causing serious vision impairment, while others go for decades without a marked change in their eyesight.

In this chapter, we will look at the three types of ARMD and chart likely changes in symptoms and in vision. What we cannot do with any certainty is assign a probable time frame to changes.

DRY ARMD

Eighty-five to 90 percent of those diagnosed with early-stage ARMD remain with that static diagnosis, and with very much the same vision, for their lifetime. It is entirely possible that the early stage of ARMD may be the only stage you ever experience, unless you live well beyond your 100th birthday. As a result, your vision may be impacted, but not very dramatically.

The typical complaint of patients with dry ARMD is mild to moderate loss of visual acuity. Details are less apparent than they once were, and blurriness is an intermittent problem. Once a doctor has told you that you have macular degeneration, you may begin to obsess about the prospects of deteriorating vision. It is important to remain attentive to changes in your vision that persist for more than a day or two, and to changes that seem to follow a pattern. But it is not constructive to become so preoccupied with the possible prospect of macular blindness that you create unwarranted concern or overreact to normal variations in your visual abilities.

Patients frequently ask me how much deterioration to expect, and I am hard-pressed to answer. The impact of age-related macular degeneration varies enormously from patient to patient and is not always measurable on a standard eye chart. It is even possible to be diagnosed with ARMD and still see the same lines on the eye chart. If your vision was 20/40 one year before the diagnosis, it may well be the same one year after it. But the letters on the chart will probably be less distinct, and you will likely have to put more effort into reading each line.

It is also possible that you see differently than your doctor thinks you see. This phenomenon is attributable to the peculiarities of vision, which is largely a matter of personal experience, not clinical measurement. It is also a result of the fact that however much we know about ARMD today that we didn't know yesterday, we still lack much vital information.

Marion Gould was diagnosed with macular degeneration after complaining of difficulty reading the street signs she passed each day while commuting to and from her office. Her ophthalmologist made the diagnosis after reviewing her angiograms, which revealed several soft drusen in both eyes, drusen that were not large but were nevertheless distinctly evident. After two years, the problem seemed no better and no worse, but then she gradually became aware that she was also having difficulty reading freeway signs, with much larger lettering than ordinary street signs. When she consulted her ophthalmologist and took the standard eye chart exam, her visual acuity was recorded as 20/30 in one eye and 20/60 in the other. This was, in fact, a slight improvement from her last exam, when the measurements were 20/40 and 20/60, respectively. Marion's angiograms showed a static condition with no bleeding—indeed, no detectable change whatsoever.

"I felt cheated," she recalls with irony. "My sight was clearly worse. Obviously I don't have to read the street signs or the freeway signs on the same route I've driven for twelve years, but I know that when I look at them, they are less visible to me than they were even a few months ago. Even if medical science has no cure for ARMD, my doctor should at least be able to supply the data that would confirm the deterioration I've experienced."

Marion Gould, like many others, doesn't see as well as she used to, but her doctor could not have determined that fact without her telling him, and she is unable to explain it. She feels both the distress of decreasing sight and the absence of support from the medical community, which can't even confirm her own reality. Regrettably, Marion's experience is not unusual. It derives from the fact that ARMD produces changes that are sometimes permanent, sometime fleeting, but not necessarily measurable. It is analogous to the ups and downs arthritis sufferers experience, when one day the pain is intense, while other days it is barely noticeable. What makes the down days more frightening for ARMD patients is the knowledge that the disease can and does progress in unpredictable and unpreventable ways. If science were able to anticipate the deterioration of one's vision with certainty, a degree of fear would be eliminated. But unexpected changes are the nature of this disease, including temporary improvement of vision and, in some rare cases, improvement that is lasting.

Late-Stage Dry ARMD

Late stage is a medical term used to define the end stage of a disease; in the case of ARMD it implies a drastic vision loss. Late-stage dry ARMD is a rare condition, affecting only about 1 to 2 percent of the patient population severely affected by both dry and wet ARMD. The vision loss is the result of a progressive thinning, or atrophy, of the retina. The etiology of this form of ARMD is currently unknown, but speculation centers on the possible loss of adequate blood supply to the retina. In some cases the decreased blood supply may be the result of cardiovascular risk factors such as atherosclerosis or hypertension.

WET ARMD

If you have been diagnosed with wet macular degeneration, there is generally a progressive loss of vision. Patients with choroidal neovascularization typically will experience a hole or distortion in their vision. For example, the word *FRAGILE* will appear distorted in a very particular way: One letter will be missing, and the more you concentrate on trying to bring that letter into focus, the more elusive it becomes.

FRAGILE looks like FR GILE

But if you stop looking for the *A* and focus instead on the *L,* the word begins to look like this:

FRAGI E

The extent of the disease will determine the degree of visual impairment, but only up to a point. Two patients with similar retinal problems will not necessarily "see" the same way. It is also possible that the explanation for the disparity may not be entirely physical. One patient may be more accepting of his condition, develop a greater degree of dependence on his good eye, or not really strain to see new things. If your daily routine is comparatively standardized, if you are not in the position of having to cope independently in new situations all the time, you will probably be less aware of impaired vision. If you don't do a lot of "close work"—needlepoint, fly-tying, or reading—compromised central vision may not be as significant to you and therefore won't seem as serious.

Late-Stage Wet ARMD

This form of wet ARMD occurs in about 9 to 12 percent of all the patients who are severely affected by ARMD. One of its characteristics is that the missing-letter effect can be even more pronounced, so that when you look directly at people, their facial characteristics all but vanish. This is attributable to retinal damage, specifically the scars left from one or more leaking blood vessels.

Progression of the disease seems to be dependent upon the type, size, and location of the blood vessels. Seriously diminished central vision can and does progress in both eyes of some patients to the point where they are "legally blind." If your vision, as measured on the standardized eye chart, is 20/200 or worse, you fit the legal description. This means that what a person with normal eyesight sees at 200 feet away, you must bring to less than 20 feet to see clearly. It does not mean that you are totally blind, but rather that you are "legally" blind.

Distortion is another common complaint in those with late-stage ARMD. Often the distortion is characterized by undulating forms where you know there ought to be straight lines. Venetian blinds look wavy across the span of a window, and fence posts appear to be swaggering across a field.

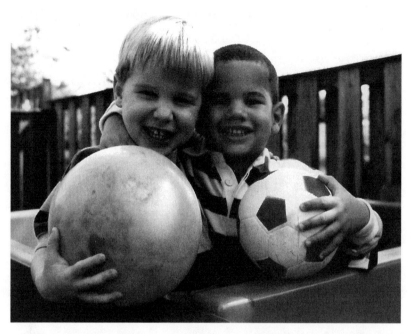

View of faces as seen normally (*above*) and with vision distorted by
late-stage wet ARMD (*below*).
(*National Eye Institute, National Institutes of Health*)

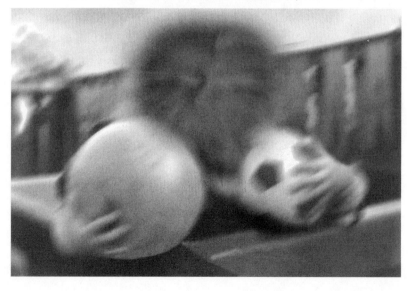

Even imaginary visions, or phantom visions as they are called, can occur. A rare experience known as the "Charles Bonnet" syndrome is sometimes reported. This syndrome is named after an eighteenth-century Swiss man who kept a written record of the phantom visions experienced by a family member whose sight had badly deteriorated. He then kept a diary of his own imaginings, as his sight, too, grew worse late in life. The phenomenon of phantom visions was named for him and his meticulous records, the first written history of the experience.

While some people tell of very specific sights—cornfields, for example, or porpoises or even relatives—most often a phantom vision is experienced as a sudden, startling shadow. "I thought I saw something," patients say, remembering when they were frightened by a figure at the window or had the feeling that someone was leaning over the back of the chair in which they were sitting.

Science has no explanation for these imaginary visions, but based on the reports from patients with ARMD, we have no reason to doubt their existence. Though they can be unpleasant and sometimes alarming, they are not, per se, a sign of advancing disease. Some people might even be described as the fortunate few; they report seeing beauty and artistic visions where those with "normal sight" see nothing.

PIGMENT EPITHELIAL DETACHMENT (PED)

Those who have been diagnosed with PED generally experience vision problems that mimic those of late-stage wet ARMD patients. Blank spots or visual distortions, and sometimes both, are the most common complaints. If the condition is severe, the blank spots in one's vision are more dominant than the clear peripheral vision; the clinical description may not be "total" loss of vision, but the experience can be perilously close.

RETENTION OF PERIPHERAL VISION

Although we don't know as much as we would like about the time frame of ARMD or the extent of vision loss, we do know what virtually every patient can expect to retain. Peripheral vision will never be lost as a direct result of this disease. Every patient will retain the ability to see things on the periphery of his or her world and can learn to use that type of vision to enhance what is still visible. This is not the same, nor anywhere near as satisfying, as retaining one's central vision, but it should be of some comfort even to those with late-stage wet ARMD.

Surprising as it may seem, patients with retinitis pigmentosa, a disease that causes loss of one's peripheral vision while central vision is preserved, often are more visually disabled than ARMD patients. The reason for this is that your peripheral vision is essential for simply moving about, whether across the room or across the continent. For example, without peripheral vision a person can easily step off the curb in front of an oncoming car because even a car is virtually invisible. Thus it is important to remember that ARMD very rarely results in total blindness or total dependence. And your world will never be completely dark.

WATCH OUT FOR OTHER
EYE PROBLEMS

Whether you have ARMD or not, you can develop other forms of retinal problems. Floaters and light flashes can be experienced by people with damage to the peripheral retina from age-related changes in the vitreous of the eye.

Ben Martin was actually anticipating eye problems as he approached his fiftieth birthday, because there was a history of age-related macular degeneration in his family, both on his mother's side and his father's. He was conscientious about going for yearly eye exams, which showed no clinical signs of any macular disease, and his only vision problem was easily corrected with typical "over-forty" reading glasses, which he bought in a supermarket for fifteen dollars. Given his family history, Ben knew what signs to watch for and checked his Amsler Grid regularly. He never experienced the "classic" symptoms and so ignored what fleeting signs of change he actually did experience.

Ben took his wife, Margey, to Hawaii for their twenty-fifth wedding anniversary and settled down on the beach for ten days of pure relaxation. Swathed in both suntan lotion and bug spray to protect his sensitive skin, Ben was vaguely annoyed at the bugs that nevertheless seemed ever present. Margey was aware of them, too, but found them nowhere near as troublesome as Ben did.

"Then one day on the tennis court," Ben recalls, "I decided that either the bugs had slowed their flight to the speed of gliders, or there were small, dark tennis balls mysteriously being lobbed over the net somehow. I was so prepared for the loss of central vision, so fanatic about checking that the strings on my racket always looked straight and regular, that I was caught completely off-guard by 'floaters.' After all, we were vacationing, enjoying the trip of a lifetime. As concerned as I always was about the possibility of ARMD, I failed to pay attention to any signs of eye problems that I wasn't already expecting."

Next came light flashes and headaches, symptoms that Ben wrote off to excessive tropical heat, and maybe even to those wonderful Mai-tais with decorative gardenias. When he and Margey returned from their trip, Ben continued to see floaters and flashing lights, but he did not visit the ophthalmologist because he could still explain away these symptoms and they weren't what he had prepared for.

When Ben finally scheduled an eye exam, he learned he had a tear in the peripheral retina, which could have been detected earlier had Ben not been focusing exclusively on signs of ARMD. Any change in your vision whatsoever should be brought to the attention of your ophthalmologist, even if your central vision is stable.

BE YOUR OWN BEST EXPERT

It certainly is desirable to think that the minute a new treatment is clinically proven to be effective in the management of ARMD, your doctor's first telephone call, upon hearing the news, will be to you. But your doctor may have hundreds of ARMD patients who all deserve to be called at the same moment. And if you live in a small rural town and spend much time in the world of cyberspace, you may even know more than your own doctor does about ARMD treatment experiments going on around the globe. The days are long gone when the doctor was the expert and the patient the dutiful listener.

You should always feel free to raise questions with your ophthalmologist concerning trials you've read about in the newspaper or information that has appeared on the Internet. It may be that your doctor hasn't heard about some obscure clue that researchers have uncovered somewhere in the world. It's also possible that your doctor knows a good deal about the research and that a press release you read in the newspaper was overly optimistic.

In any event, your best hope in dealing with ARMD is good information. Get it where you can and discuss it fully with your treating physician.

PART TWO

Treatment Options

6

⚜

Therapies for
Dry ARMD

If you have no particular difficulties with your vision and if, during a routine visit to the ophthalmologist, you learn you have drusen or are diagnosed with dry ARMD, there is no reason to react with alarm. Your condition may not change for the next fifty years. While you may be one of the millions of Americans who are affected by ARMD, you may also be one of the lucky individuals who are asymptomatic and remain so forever. Even when you are told about the drusen in response to complaints about poor eyesight, you may not encounter extensive vision problems if fluorescein angiography determines that there are no abnormal blood vessels in your retina.

Although there are no scientifically proven medications or treatment procedures for mild, dry ARMD, preventive care as well as lifestyle changes will almost certainly retard disease progression. This news is not

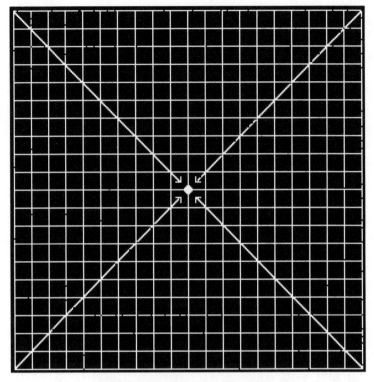

Black-on-white Amsler Grid.
(Macular Degeneration Foundation)

always welcomed by patients, many of whom would prefer a dramatic, all-purpose, quick, and easy cure to having to adopt a healthier lifestyle. But the truth of the matter is that healthy living *is* the best treatment today for dry ARMD, and that every patient has the capacity to make the necessary changes right away.

It is also essential that patients with dry ARMD exercise constant vigilance in monitoring their vision. They need to have ophthalmic checkups at six-month intervals, and if they detect any obvious changes in vision, they shouldn't wait for the next checkup but schedule an appointment with the eye doctor immediately.

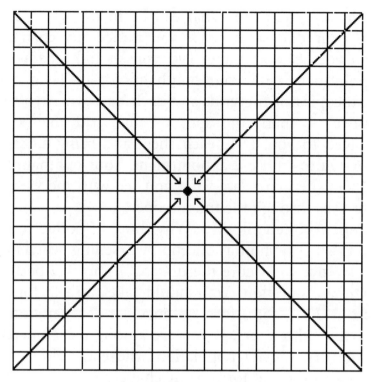

White-on-black Amsler Grid.
(Macular Degeneration Foundation)

MONITORING YOUR STATUS WITH THE AMSLER GRID

The Amsler Grid is a tool that should be used on a daily basis to screen for any subtle changes in your vision, changes that may not be obvious as you go about the course of your normal activities. It is designed to isolate your capacity to "fixate," that is, your ability to use your central, or macular, vision. Two types of grids are available: One has white lines on a black background; the other, black lines on a white background. Most patients find the black background easier to work with.

This is a quick test that can be incorporated easily into your daily routine. If you notice any change in what you see with either eye, you should schedule an appointment with your ophthalmologist. Then make photocopies of the grid, and each day, when you test your eyes, mark the spot on the grid that seems changed to you. Date each sheet and bring all sheets with you to your eye appointment. Your ophthalmologist can then correlate what you see with the views of your eyes through the microscope.

Patients often ask me, "Why should I bother to take a test that may show a condition worsening, when medical science can't cure the disease?" This is a perfectly legitimate question. You should take the test for two reasons. First, some forms of macular degeneration are treatable with lasers. If you are among the 10 percent of the dry ARMD population whose condition progresses to the wet form, your chances of being treated effectively by laser therapy are improved if you are alert to changes in your vision and are able to communicate them immediately to your ophthalmologist. (See chapter 7 for a detailed discussion of laser therapy.)

The second reason for taking the test is that it might reveal the presence of a condition unrelated to your macular degeneration, and that problem might be both treatable and curable. When you have been diagnosed with a progressive eye disease, it is perfectly logical to conclude that any deterioration in your sight is merely a confirmation of the original diagnosis. But this is not always true. The experience of my coauthor, Joan Snyder, illustrates the point perfectly.

Having sensed the appearance of a blank spot or

some indistinct "hole" in her vision, Joan consulted an ophthalmologist, who diagnosed her condition as age-related macular degeneration. The information she received was depressingly incomplete, and she was told that the best she could hope for was a very slow progression of the disease. A second opinion confirmed the diagnosis, and Joan geared herself to accept the inevitability of slowly failing eyesight. As the blank spot worsened, she consulted a third doctor to see if she might hear a more hopeful report. This doctor told Joan that her visual symptoms were the result of an incipient hole in the retina of her right eye, and that they could be corrected with surgery. The macular degeneration diagnosis was partially accurate, because in the left eye, she did indeed have drusen. But the blank spot in the right eye, where no drusen were present, was attributable to an altogether different macular problem.

You are surely the best person to evaluate your own eyesight, but your doctor is the best person to diagnose the reason for any changes in your vision. Age-related macular degeneration does not preclude the possibility of other problems, and changes in your central vision should never be automatically attributed to ARMD.

The Amsler Grid is the most effective tool we have for early detection of changes in vision. Use it every day of your life. Wallet-sized Amsler Grids can be obtained from Lighthouse International (see the "Resources" section), from most ophthalmologists, or downloaded from a number of different Web sites, including this one: www.eyesight.org.

How to Use the Amsler Grid

The Amsler Grid is easy to use. Take the test for each eye individually by covering one eye at a time. Be sure to hold the grid at exactly the same distance, approximately fifteen inches from your eye, in every test. Focus on the dot in the center of the grid. Are the lines blurry or gray? Do pieces of the grid disappear when you focus intently on that spot alone?

Be sure to examine the grid in bright light with your reading glasses *on*. It will seem blurry if you need corrective lenses and don't use them to read the grid.

PREVENTIVE CARE

In addition to checking your vision with the Amsler Grid, you need to take certain precautions to lower your risk of further eye deterioration. These include protecting your eyes from bright sunlight and following a diet that is low in fat.

Protection Against Ultraviolet Light

Research is currently being conducted to determine whether exposure to a great deal of bright sunlight speeds up macular deterioration or even causes it. The results of the studies are incomplete, but there is reason to believe that protecting your eyes from bright light with sunglasses, preferably those designed to filter out blue and ultraviolet (UV) light, is a wise precaution.

This belief is based on our knowledge that cataract removal allows more light to reach the retina and increases one's chances of developing different types of macular disease.

Light can damage both the lens in the eye and the retina. Damage to the lens generally results in cataract formation. After a cataract blocks the vision of the eye, it may reduce the amount of light that can then enter. But for those who spend a great deal of time outdoors in bright light, it's likely that the retina is already damaged from light exposure before cataracts form. This is why studies reveal that patients with cataracts have a greater incidence of ARMD than those without cataracts. Moreoever, once cataracts have formed and then been removed, ARMD may actually accelerate, a result of either increased light exposure or the inflammation often associated with cataract surgery.*

Some doctors believe that during certain periods of our lives we are particularly vulnerable to damage from light exposure. This theory holds that before age thirty, and after fifty, we are most susceptible to retina damage from solar radiation. In early life, the lens is most transparent, allowing the most light to impact the retina. In later life, the melanin and antioxidants in the retina that protect it from light damage may dissipate. (Antioxidants are substances that are thought to reduce cellular destruction of all kinds, eliminating the "free radicals" that circulate in our bodies when cells have

*R. Klein, B. E. Klein, S. C. Jensen, and K. J. Cruickshanks, "The Relationship of Ocular Factors to the Incidence and Progression of Age-Related Maculopathy," *Archives of Ophthalmology* 116, no. 4 (April 1998):506–13.

died.) The migration of many seniors to sunny climates may actually exacerbate the problem of age-related vision problems, including age-related macular degeneration.

An ordinary pair of sunglasses often blocks out as little as 60 percent of the sun's harmful rays. It is advisable to purchase glasses that block out 100 percent of UV-A and UV-B sun rays. They should also filter out at least 85 percent of the blue-violet sun rays that some practitioners believe may accelerate the development of age-related macular degeneration by producing free radicals in the retina. Because sunglasses have become such an important fashion accessory, you should be able to find a stylish pair for very little money that also protects your eyesight and retards macular degeneration.

Alcohol Consumption

Moderate alcohol consumption seems to have some beneficial effect on cardiovascular disease, and through a similar mechanism, it could have a beneficial impact on ARMD. In one study, the first National Health and Nutrition Examination Survey, researchers discovered that even after adjusting survey results for age, sex, income, history of congestive heart failure, and hypertension, wine seemed to have a positive influence. Those who consumed wine had a lower incidence of ARMD than those who were completely abstemious. Researchers speculated that their findings might be explained by the high concentrations of antioxidant phenolic compounds in red wine. There have been few epidemiological studies, however, that purport to examine the relationship between alcohol consumption and ARMD exclusively. The most recent study that did focus on this one variable found no change in the incidence of ARMD with increasing alcohol consumption.*

Low-Fat Diet

A good diet generally produces a healthy body, and it is obvious that if you have any disease, including ARMD, it is important to eat properly to give yourself as much nutritional benefit as possible. For example, we all know that a diet low in saturated fats is conducive to good health, and it may be particularly important for ARMD patients and those who are at risk for the disease based on their family history. A diet deficient in omega-3 fats (such as those from cold water fish) and one high in saturated fats (such as those in butter or animal fat) has been shown to result in impairment of the retinal functioning in rodents. We also know that omega-3 fats are beneficial to cardiovascular and ocular systems, suggesting not only that a low-fat diet is important, but that avoiding certain fats while including others is the appropriate dietary strategy.

Two studies looked at the association between dietary fat intake and ARMD, and both suggested that fat intake—especially saturated fat intake—is positively related to the disease.† The degree of correlation is still

*U. A. Ajani et al., "A Prospective Study of Alcohol Consumption and the Risk of Age-Related Macular Degeneration," *American Epidemiology* 9, no. 3 (April 1999):172–77.
†J. A. Mares-Pearlman et al., "Dietary Fat and Age-Related Maculopathy," *Archives of Ophthalmology* 113, no. 6 (June 1995): 743–48.

unclear, but scientific evidence clearly points to the following conclusion: Even if you have difficulty reducing the quantity of fat intake, it is wise to modify the type of fat you ingest. Both canola oil and olive oil are preferable to other liquid oils, and any liquid fat is preferable to fats that are solid at room temperature, such as lard, butter, and margarine.

VITAMINS AND NUTRITIONAL SUPPLEMENTS

Antioxidants

These substances are often reported to be the cure-all for many age-related diseases. There are a wide variety of antioxidants, and most of them are created naturally in our bodies or are ingested when we eat foods high in vitamins C, A, and E. A great deal of research interest is centered on isolating the impact of antioxidant vitamins on ARMD, and studies on each of the three major vitamins are now under way.

So far, epidemiological studies have not supported the notion that vitamin C, A, or E can play a protective role in reducing the risk of developing ARMD. One study does conclude that those who ingest higher-than-average quantities of vitamin C may have a slightly lower risk for ARMD; but this finding applies to those who consume food with high natural quantities of vitamin C, not necessarily to those who take vitamin C supplements.*

*Eye Disease Case-Control Study Group, J. M. Seddon et al., "Dietary Carotenoids, Vitamins A, C, and E and Advanced Age-

One can purchase synthetic antioxidants without a prescription wherever vitamins are sold, but scientific studies have not proven the efficacy of antioxidants in treating macular degeneration once the eyes are damaged. Megadoses of vitamins can be dangerous. In fact, high doses of vitamin A may actually accelerate the progression of some types of cancer. For example, beta-carotene taken at what the medical profession calls "pharmacological levels" (that is, doses above the Recommended Daily Allowance) actually increases the incidence of lung cancer in cigarette smokers.* Thus the notion that these agents are totally harmless is false.

There are isolated research articles, however, suggesting a connection between certain antioxidants and healthy eyes. The Age-Related Eye Disease Study (AREDS), conducted by the National Institutes of Health, evaluated, in randomized clinical trials, the effects of pharmacological doses of antioxidants and zinc on the progression of ARMD. (We'll take a closer look at zinc later in this chapter.) Approximately 5,000 patients were enrolled in the study, which began in 1994 and was completed in 2000, to determine the impact of various combinations of vitamin supplements. Patients at higher risk of developing vision loss due to ARMD were randomly placed in four groups: antioxidant vitamins, zinc, antioxidant vitamins and zinc, and placebo.

Related Macular Degeneration," *JAMA* 272, no. 18 (November 9, 1994):1413–20.
*D. Albanes et al. "Alpha-Tocopherol and Beta-Carotene Supplements and Lung Cancer Incidence in the Alpha Tocopherol, Beta-Carotene Cancer Prevention Study: Effects of Base-line Characteristics and Study Compliance," *Journal of the National Cancer Institute* (November 6, 1996), 88 (21):1560–70.

Patients at low risk of developing visual loss through ARMD were assigned to two groups: high-dose antioxidants and placebo. Until these findings are published, I recommend that you consume plenty of fruits and vegetables to obtain adequate antioxidant protection.

Carotenoids

Carotenoids are pigments found in plants that have the ability to absorb visible light. Fruits and vegetables are the major sources of carotenoids, and studies have recently been published that focus on the potential antioxidant function of specific carotenoids found in the eye. In particular, lutein and zeaxanthin were associated with reduced risk of ARMD, meaning that the population that had a higher dietary intake of foods with lutein and zeaxanthin had fewer cases of ARMD. This study indicates that eating leafy green vegetables five or more times a week—vegetables such as spinach, collard greens, kale, mustard, or turnip greens—results in a markedly reduced risk of ARMD.*

It is faulty logic to conclude that lutein or zeaxanthin can cure ARMD or even retard its progression, but it is not necessarily illogical to believe that there is a connection between levels of these carotenoids and ocular health. Spinach is one of the best sources of lutein, and preferable, in my judgment, to powdered lutein supplements, which are, however, available without prescrip-

*Eye Disease Case-Control Study Group, J. M. Seddon et al., "Dietary Carotenoids, Vitamins A, C, and E, and Advanced Age-Related Macular Degeneration," *JAMA* 272, no. 18 (November 9, 1994):1413–20.

tion. Other foods with high lutein content include egg yolks, kiwi fruit, and apricots.

Zinc

Much has been written in alternative medicine publications about the value of zinc for macular degeneration patients, and indeed, there is a connection between zinc and healthy eyes. The retina has a high concentration of zinc, though science is unable to totally define the role this trace element plays in retinal functioning. Some studies do show a correlation between zinc and less deterioration for ARMD patients; others do not. There is, to date, little research supporting the notion that massive doses of zinc are helpful in curing the disease. In fact, too much zinc in the diet can actually be harmful. Adequate zinc is generally provided by a daily multivitamin and, more important, by a diet high in fruits and vegetables. In my view, dietary zinc is preferable to zinc supplements because it prevents excessive dosage and promotes attention to proper nutritional balance in all meal planning.

7

Medical Treatments for Wet ARMD

Although wet ARMD is far less prevalent than its dry form, it is considerably more debilitating. In virtually every case, patients experience a serious loss of central vision and may encounter other problems as well, including distorted straight lines and a loss of color awareness.

THE PROS AND CONS OF LASER THERAPY

Laser therapy for retinal problems (known as photocoagulation) involves the use of a high-energy light, a laser beam, which turns to heat when it hits the parts of the retina to be treated. It is quite different from the corneal laser techniques used for vision correction and also from the procedure used for cataract removal. Laser therapy is applied most often in the treatment of "wet" ARMD. The laser is beamed onto the leaking blood vessels, and this action stops the bleeding or fluid leakage, forming a scar over that spot in the retina.

Although laser therapy is not considered the customary treatment for dry ARMD, it is being used on an experimental basis by some retinal specialists to treat the drusen before any new blood vessels have grown. Usually in these cases, the doctor has reason to anticipate that leaking blood vessels will almost surely develop. One example would be a patient whose dry ARMD progressed rapidly to wet in one eye, and who has severe drusen in the other eye.

Some of these laser experiments have proven quite effective. In fact, in most dry ARMD cases where the laser treatment has been tried, drusen have disappeared. But following laser treatment, some patients also grew new, abnormal blood vessels where previously there were none. Was the laser the cause of their growth? Might the blood vessels have grown in any event, even without laser treatment? These questions remain unanswered for the moment, and though experiments with different intensities of laser light continue, this treatment program is rarely prescribed for ordinary cases of dry macular degeneration.

Laser therapy is more likely to be offered as a treatment for wet ARMD. If the abnormal blood vessel is discovered early enough, this treatment may be helpful. The procedure is painless, generally completed within an hour, and is ordinarily conducted on an outpatient basis. One risk of laser therapy worthy of mention is excessive bleeding, which may cause other postoperative complications, though the incidence of this type of bleeding is extremely rare.

Following treatment, as noted earlier, a scar will form on the retina where the laser eliminated the abnormal blood vessel (CNV). The scar will produce a blind spot in your vision. The size, location, and number of the CNV treated by laser will determine the amount of lost vision, so it is essential to discuss with your doctor the extent of laser treatment he or she recommends.

From the patient's perspective, treatment of vessels that are near the center of the fovea but not directly under the fovea yields the most satisfactory results. The reason is that a small blind spot adjacent to the center of your vision produces a lesser disability than a blind spot directly in the center.

The objective of the laser treatment is to destroy the CNV and the associated leakage so that it will not continue to destroy ever-greater portions of your vision. There is, however, a downside to this treatment: Your vision may temporarily or permanently worsen after laser therapy because the laser scar generally is slightly larger than the original CNV. But it usually produces less severe vision loss than would have occurred ultimately had the blood vessel been left to grow unchecked.

Not all patients are appropriate candidates for this treatment, since CNV shows up in many different shapes and sizes, depending upon the patient. Which patients, then, are appropriate candidates for laser treatment? General recommendations are as follows:

- If you have a CNV that is plainly demarcated and outside the central foveal area, you may be a logical candidate for laser therapy.

- If you have a CNV that is plainly demarcated and inside the central foveal area, you may also be a candidate for laser therapy, but a less significant benefit should be expected. Although the laser treatment will significantly worsen your vision in the short term, your vision in the long run will be better than it would have been without treatment. The treatment of CNV under the fovea is controversial because, even with treatment, the outcome may be poor. Newer types of laser treatment, however, such as photodynamic therapy (see next section), may improve the outcome in this type of situation.

Follow-up studies on laser-treated ARMD patients indicate that after five years, the loss of vision was less acute than in the control group, which had no laser treatment. Nonsmokers and individuals without hypertension had a higher success rate. But much depends, too, on the location of the blood vessel being treated and the type of lesion.

Even if you are a logical candidate for laser treatment, you should be aware that it is a successful procedure in only a small portion of cases. In general, 15 percent of the patient population with wet ARMD are good candidates for the treatment in the first place, usually those with leaking blood vessels outside the fovea. In addition, these lesions or CNV must be characterized as "classic" or well defined to be treated with beneficial results. After treatment, we find that in approximately half the cases, the bleeding has stopped and the blood vessels have not grown back. From a medical perspective, this is deemed a success.

Patients who have experienced laser treatment have widely divergent views of its benefits. One offered the following comment: "I was recently diagnosed with MD, but my vision was relatively good until the doctor said, 'I am going to save your sight.' He lasered it, and his vision was made much worse. Others complain that they were surprised by the sudden loss of vision after a procedure that purported to be constructive. Disillusionment is easy to understand if the patient was not made aware of the prospective loss of sight or did not understand that the loss of vision after the surgery was the lesser of two evils; without surgery, chances are that there would have been much greater loss of vision when the disease progressed.

May Saunders had no warning of any vision problems when she realized she had lost virtually all sight in her left eye. It was not a case of gradual, progressive deterioration. "It was more like someone holding a black cue ball directly in front of my eye," she remembers. "I knew immediately the problem was serious." Her ophthalmologist advised her to do nothing about it, but when her right eye started to deteriorate, she took immediate action. "I ran to his office like a racehorse and insisted on laser treatment. I knew all about what I had to lose, both in treatment and, most probably, without it. I was determined to save whatever sight could be salvaged in my right eye, because the 20/800 I had in my left was a very clear and daily reminder of what I might have without it. I'm fortunate, because after three laser treatments, I still have 20/200 in my right eye, and far more vision than I believe I might have had otherwise."

May is a good example of a patient who is satisfied,

if not thrilled, with the results of laser therapy. One reason for her satisfaction is that she had previewed the probable downside of no treatment. Every patient must weigh a number of factors that affect his or her lifestyle in making a decision of this magnitude. Until better alternatives are offered, laser therapy may be the only treatment your ophthalmologist can provide; but this doesn't mean it is necessarily right for you. The decision must be a personal choice.

Where laser treatment *is* recommended by the retinal specialist, it should be performed by a highly experienced ophthalmologist with specialized training. As a practicing ophthalmologist, I can assure you that you should not hesitate to ask your doctor about his or her experience in treating macular degeneration patients with lasers and about the success rate following treatment. You may also want to talk to a retinal ophthalmologist who specializes in this type of treatment. Names of these specialists are available from the American Academy of Ophthalmology and the Macular Degeneration Foundation (see the "Resources" section).

EXPERIMENTAL PHOTODYNAMIC THERAPY

Photodynamic therapy (PDT) is one of the newest treatment programs for wet ARMD. Because it is so new, the treatment parameters are still being revised, but data from clinical studies suggest that the therapy is promising. The most significant feature of this treatment is that, unlike conventional laser therapy, PDT is able to treat the leaking blood vessels under the retina with less damage to surrounding tissue. Consequently, the patient's posttreatment experience is far more positive than with standard lasers.

The treatment involves the introduction of a dye into the body that accumulates in neovascular tissue, specifically in the leaking blood vessels. The dye is made up of a mixture of molecules that react to, or are activated by, light; hence it is referred to as a photosensitizer. Ordinary light normally has no effect, but light at a very specific wavelength will cause the molecules to convert to free radicals. These agents then attack the leaking blood vessels and effectively destroy them.

The effect seems to be temporary, requiring treatment every three months to prevent the blood vessels from regrowing. Vision may continue to decline, although it will quite probably do so at a slower rate than without treatment. This is the reason that PDT is insufficient as a complete cure for ARMD, even though it is one of the most promising treatments being developed at this moment.

Several pharmaceutical companies are testing different types of photosensitizers to determine which are most effective in destroying the maximum amount of unwanted vasculature with minimum effect on other tissue. How frequently, how aggressively, and how repeatedly the therapy should be conducted are all questions yet to be answered. In late 1999, members of a panel advising the Food and Drug Administration said they thought that PDT was safe and effective for treating well-defined subfoveal CNV.* They cautioned,

---

*Their comments related to PDT as conducted in studies using the photosensitizer Visudyne.

however, that the treatment provided only modest benefit for certain patients and urged the FDA to look more closely at long-term studies. Specifically, they noted what was well recognized already—that PDT cannot restore vision lost from ARMD. Final approval from the FDA was granted in April 2000, and this therapy should be available to practicing ophthalmologists during the second half of 2000.

If you do undergo PDT, you can expect a course of treatment that is similar to angiography testing, one that is both painless and noninvasive. The photosensitizing compound is injected by needle into your arm, and within minutes, the blood vessels have absorbed it. A special wavelength of light is projected into your eye, activating the chemical chain reaction. Since there is a small possibility that the compounds will be weakly activated by sunlight, patients are instructed to avoid exposure to direct sunlight for several days following treatment.

TRANSPUPILLARY THERMOTHERAPY

This technique is similar to conventional laser therapy but uses a diode laser, which can treat abnormal blood vessels with a beam of only 45° to 60°C (115° to 130°F), considerably lower than that used in a conventional laser burn. The benefit is that the lower temperature causes less collateral damage to surrounding tissue and to the retina. In a small, uncontrolled study conducted by Dr. Elias Reichel in Boston, 20 percent of the patients treated with transpupillary thermotherapy (TTT) showed improvement, and 56 percent remained stable when their condition would otherwise have been expected to deteriorate. No deleterious side effects were seen. This technique appears promising, and a randomized, clinical study is being organized to evaluate how effective the treatment might be.*

DRUG THERAPY

Patients and doctors alike are always hopeful that a "silver bullet" will be found to treat a given disease simply, effectively, and painlessly. With ARMD, not only is there no such pill, there is no existing therapy that can effectively treat the disease with a predictable, beneficial outcome. There is under study, however, an innovative approach to the management of CNV. Known as angiogenesis inhibition, this approach uses a very different premise from that on which laser therapy is based. It attempts to directly inhibit the factors that support the growth of these new blood vessels or to interfere with the growth of endothelial cells that form these vessels.

In 1992 I began to investigate drugs for potential antiangiogenic properties. I felt that any drug that had antiangiogenic activity must have left some clues in the form of side effects consistent with blood vessel inhibition. I knew that a woman taking a drug with antiangiogenic activity would likely experience disruption of her menstrual cycles, and that if she took such a drug

*E. Reichel et al., "Transpupillary Thermotherapy of Occult Subfoveal Choroidal Neovascularization in Patients with Age-Related Macular Degeneration," *Ophthalmology* 106, no. 10 (October 1999):1908–14.

New Antiangiogenic Agents in Ocular Trials

Company	Compound
Alcon	Anecortave Acetate—Periocular
Agouron	AG3340—Oral
Genentech	Human FAb antiVEGF—Intravitreal
Lilly	LY333531—Oral
NeXstar	NX1838—Intravitreal

when she was pregnant, it might cause abnormal fetal development and subsequent birth defects. With this thought in mind, I searched the literature for cases where drugs had caused these outcomes, either blocked menstrual cycles or birth defects.

Very few drugs had been reported to cause these side effects, but one that did, and resulted in widely publicized heartbreak to mothers all over the world, was thalidomide. Although the drug had been introduced in the late 1950s as a sedative for pregnant women, it was later found to cause irreparable damage to the limbs of newborns. I thought that if I were able to unlock the secrets of how thalidomide had resulted in such potent harm to fetuses, the very same mechanism might be reapplied in a therapeutic manner, to inhibit the growth of abnormal blood vessels in ARMD or in arresting malignant tumors.

A causal link for this catastrophe was not clear to my colleagues and me until we found that thalidomide prevented the development of newly stimulated blood vessels, which may have damaged the formation of developing limbs. This connection led us to believe that thalidomide might well be effective in preventing the growth of *improper* vasculature in the eyes, in much the same way that it had damaged *proper* vasculature in the fetus. After exhaustive research, we confirmed our hypothesis in 1994 and published our results: Not only did thalidomide prevent the development of newly stimulated blood vessels in the eyes of treated animals, it had no impact on the normal, mature blood vessels.

The discovery of thalidomide as an angiogenesis inhibitor led us to conduct ongoing studies beginning in 1994, which follow two groups of patients: those with leaking blood vessels that cannot be treated with lasers or photodynamic therapy, and a second group that had undergone laser treatment. In this second sample we have been trying to determine if thalidomide, taken in carefully prescribed small doses, can limit the recurrence of treated blood vessels and prevent the formation of new ones. Unfortunately, early results have suggested that the drug's side effects—sedation and constipation—are not well tolerated in an elderly population at the dosage levels tested (200 mg/day). Although thalidomide may not prove to be the optimal inhibitor for ARMD, other drugs may. For a list of companies conducting ocular trials with other compounds, see the table on page 87.

Some of the latest and most promising work being done in the field of antiangiogenic agents is that of Dr. Judah Folkman. While Dr. Folkman's work is directed at inhibiting newly grown blood vessels in tumors, the findings can be extrapolated to the treatment of other abnormally growing vessels, such as those seen in ARMD. He observed that patients with cancerous tumors often have them removed successfully, only to endure subsequent explosive growth of metastasis. Trying to understand why this might occur, Folkman theorized that the primary tumor that was removed must have contained some control factor that had been suppressing the growth of other tumors. In fact, that is exactly what his investigatory team found: an angiogenesis inhibitor known as angiostatin. When purified, not only can angiostatin suppress the growth of the secondary tumors, it can be used in higher doses to inhibit the growth of the primary tumor itself. The same substance, and one very much like it called endostatin, may be expected to be potentially effective in suppressing certain types of neovascularization seen in ARMD.

The investigatory work being done in this area holds great promise for cancer patients. If trials prove promising for the treatment of malignancies, trials for the treatment of ARMD will be initiated. The scientific approach underlying angiogenesis is totally innovative; it represents, in effect, a new way of seeing a perplexing medical problem rather than the mere application of a new therapy. As such, the approach offers a thrilling opportunity to medical researchers seeking creative new avenues to heal their patients and a whole new realm of hope for those afflicted with disease.

8

Alternative Therapies

There is often an implicit cold war of sorts between "conservatives" who believe that modern medicine and scientific research will reveal all the answers to our health problems, and those who have embraced "progressive" new-age remedies based on ancient tradition.

As a doctor, I have been trained to put my trust in science. Searching for cures for this troublesome disease, I tend to be skeptical of anecdotal evidence that has not stood up to independent scientific study, and I can't recommend any therapy, conventional or alternative, where sufficient scientific proof has not been accumulated. My coauthor, however, is not a physician, and like many people, she is first and foremost a patient anxious for help. Her notion of whom and what to trust is broader than mine and reflects a philosophy that scientific proof is less important than effective results on an individual patient basis. Ultimately, each person must judge for himself or herself whether the therapies discussed in this chapter are worthy of consideration.

In alternative health systems, particular emphasis is placed on treating the person as a whole. Practitioners reason that body parts are not separately functioning units except in the context of academic science, and that treatments that care for the whole person—both the mind and the body—are always most effective, regardless of the specific complaint. Another core belief of most alternative therapy proponents is that the therapies are primarily effective with patients who are "activists," those who, with tools put at their disposal, are prepared to pick them up and use them. In the words of Meir Schneider, founder of the School of Self-Healing in San Francisco, "Conviction creates the cure."

The array of alternative therapies is vast, but those that are most often discussed in conjunction with ARMD include Eastern treatments such as acupuncture, spiritual disciplines such as meditation, and body work such as yoga or massage. Several programs include more than one of these approaches, and quite a few include the use of microstimulation of the areas around the eye. There is also a controversial treatment that is a system of blood filtration.

MICROCURRENT STIMULATION

One area of exploration that has received considerable attention from alternative therapy advocates is microcurrent stimulation. Some patients have reported not only better visual acuity but improved color perception after treatment. This technique is a noninvasive procedure in which electrical stimulation is applied to areas around the eye with a lightweight, handheld machine.

Speculation is that the improvement in visual acuity reported by some ARMD patients results from improved blood flow to the macula, or possibly from enhancement of the transport mechanism that brings required nutrients into the cones and removes waste products from them.

The hardware used in the treatment is a TENS unit (for transcutaneous electrical nerve stimulation), a simple piece of equipment currently approved by the FDA for use by orthopedic surgeons and sports medicine doctors in the treatment of chronic back and limb pain. It is also used by some plastic surgeons to accelerate wound healing after skin grafts. Several scientific studies by cardiologists have demonstrated that TENS significantly relieves chronic angina symptoms and improves blood flow in patients with extensive heart blood vessel blockages that are not correctable by surgery.

Dr. Joel Rossen of MicroStim Technology Incorporated is widely acknowledged as the "inventor" of hardware for use in microcurrent therapy. He began using the technique over twenty years ago for the treatment of pain. Some types of pain, he theorized, were not from a specific injury but from an energy imbalance that could be corrected by electrical stimulation. His successful experiments in this area led him to work with ophthalmologists and homeopaths and other alternative healers, who saw the impact of microcurrent stimulation on many who underwent treatment. At the present time, the TENS unit is approved by the FDA for use only under the supervision of, and with the prescription of, a licensed physician.

Microcurrent stimulation is purported to benefit patients with dry ARMD. There is no data to suggest that it can inhibit the wet form. However, a few ophthalmologists using it with patients who experienced a macular bleed suggest an accelerated reabsorption of blood and subsequent clearing of some central vision. The clinical significance of this observation is not clear, but more rapid and complete clearing of blood after a macular bleed may result in less scarring and thus less vision loss.

Currently, there are several small studies under way to determine if microcurrent stimulation can improve the vision of patients with dry and wet ARMD, with a large, controlled, clinical trial planned to begin early in 2000. Until the results of these studies are known, I do not recommend that microcurrent stimulation be used outside the clinical trial. At this writing, one physician conducting a trial is Dr. George Khouri of West Palm Beach, Florida. Other trials can be located by accessing the FDA Web site or by contacting MicroStim Technology Incorporated (see "Resources" section).

Anna, a patient who received a treatment in a South Dakota clinic, reports that she was helped significantly. After two treatments a day for three days and another treatment on the fourth, she went home with a handheld unit powered by a nine-volt battery. She describes the procedure she follows at home: "Two probes are attached to the unit. I place one small probe in my hand while holding conductive gel, and place the other probe, a Q-Tip saturated in conductive gel, against my eyelid. It is absolutely painless and feels like a very small twitch on the eye. It takes me twenty minutes to give myself a treatment, which I do every other day."

RHEOTHERAPY

This is a system of blood filtration known as apheresis that removes high-molecular-weight proteins and lipoproteins from the blood. The procedure is used in other areas of medicine, such as in the treatment of patients with multiple myeloma, who may exhibit what's known as a "hyperviscosity syndrome," a condition in which excess proteins are present in the blood. In ophthalmology, RheoTherapy is a subject of controversy in both the legal and medical communities at this time. There is, in my judgment, limited scientific evidence that the treatment is effective in treating ARMD and very limited support for the hypothesis that it can cure this condition.

A group of German doctors were the first to test this system of blood filtration on patients with ARMD. They treated ten patients while ten untreated patients served as a control group. Recently, they reported their finding: There was an improvement of 1.1 lines on the eye chart in the treated patients as compared with a loss of 0.6 lines in the untreated patients. Although the results appear to suggest a positive effect, accepted scientific protocol would call for verification of these results with controlled studies based on *hundreds* of patients. Moreover, the variable range of results (or the standard deviation, in more scientific terms) also suggests that larger numbers of patients will be needed before conclusions about the treatment's efficacy can be drawn.

When RheoTherapy was available in Florida, a number of people with ARMD tried the therapy. Although some of them experienced no improvement in their visual acuity or their color perception, others, such as the writer Carolyn See, reported very favorable results. Having tried conventional therapies with limited results, she decided to experiment with RheoTherapy even though, as she says, "I had no hope at all that it would work." To her surprise, she was impressed by her results and by those of others with whom she chatted at the clinic. True, neither she nor the administrators of this therapy have scientifically documented proof that this treatment is effective. But for Carolyn See, only one reality is important: Before her RheoTherapy, she could not see well enough to drive; after her treatment, she could.

As of early 2000, the treatment is no longer available in the United States and is offered, to my knowledge, only in Germany. A clinical trial in Germany is in the planning stages, and if you want to experiment with this treatment, I advise you to participate in this study or another one like it, but not to experiment outside a clinical trial.

ACUPUNCTURE AND ACUPRESSURE

Some patients with ARMD have tried acupuncture, both with the traditional needles inserted in the skin and with "electronic" needles. The latter do not puncture the skin but emit a very mild electric stimulation when placed on the surface of the skin. In Western medical science, few studies have been conducted on how or why this procedure works, but Eastern medicine has used the technique for centuries with documented results.

Acupressure is a related science that focuses on the

same meridian system, or "map of points," on the body, each of which corresponds to a precise organ or a general area. Where acupuncturists use very fine needles (which most subjects say they don't even feel) to access these points, therapists practicing acupressure use pressure, more like massage. The eyes, for example, correspond to points on the second and third fingers, also on the second and third toes. "Unlocking" or "redirecting" the energy flows in these centers is, according to holistic practitioners and many of their devoted clients, effective in improving vision.

Dr. Peggy Rollo, a physician whose practice is centered on the plant remedies of naturopathy, is licensed to practice acupuncture in Oregon. She believes that traditional acupuncture, electronic needle acupuncture, and acupressure can all be effective in treating ARMD, though in many cases she also prescribes plant remedies such as bilberry. Asked which of the three meridian-based therapies is the most effective for ARMD, Dr. Rollo replies that the answer depends upon the specific patient and his or her response to each technique. Each individual reacts differently to conventional medications, and it should be assumed that every patient has a unique response to alternative therapies as well.

YOGA, MASSAGE, AND OTHER BODY WORK

Yoga, as a combined form of relaxation and exercise, is an ancient practice and an integral part of many Eastern cultural traditions. In the past two decades, it has gained a considerable following in the United States. While there are many different forms of yoga, some far more strenuous than others, all are designed to relax the practitioner and to induce a feeling of overall good health.

Massage is another technique that produces the same effect. In itself, massage is not suggested as a therapy to cure or even retard progressive macular disease, but it is recommended by holistic practitioners as a stress-relieving therapy. Because the body's normal reaction to stress is to gear up to "overdrive," the weakest link in the system—in this case, your eyes—is taxed even more heavily, when clearly what's needed is less use and less strain on this weakened link.

According to Meir Schneider, "The bottom line with macular degeneration is relaxation and more relaxation." His holistic program, derived largely from his own very impressive recovery from "legal" blindness, is based on massage, which relaxes the muscles that control the eyes, and on a number of exercises that strengthen these muscles.

Some of his strengthening exercises are closely related to the "Bates Method," a system articulated around the turn of the nineteenth century by an ophthalmologist named William Bates. This methodology has evolved into a series of applications principally designed to improve "weak" eyes, particularly myopic eyes, but the original Bates philosophy included a great deal of visualization and relaxation work applicable to all eye problems, including macular degeneration. This aspect of the Bates system has been incorporated into Schneider's unique program, which has, according to anecdotal reports, helped many people.

At the age of twenty-eight, Ellen Carter was diagnosed with "juvenile" macular degeneration, a disease related to ARMD. Since she was a psychotherapist, and had acquired her own training as a conventional physician, she naturally turned to traditional Western medicine for treatment. Every ophthalmologist she consulted, however, told her that there was no treatment, and that she should prepare for eventual blindness. "But I never believed it," she says. "I simply never believed I would not see, no matter how expert my doctors were in their field."

Ellen had an intuitive sense that her diet was part of the problem, and she began to be much more careful about eliminating sugar and eating mostly vegetables. She also turned to acupuncture and then to Meir Schneider's body work at the School for Self-Healing. She spent three to four hours each day at the center working on changing her motor-perceptual skills, then returned to her hotel room at night to complete her homework, a lengthy and rigorous routine of eye exercises. She flew back to her home on the East Coast two weeks later with vision that had improved from 20/100 to 20/40.

Does Ellen think that everyone who undergoes this type of therapy will see the improvement that she did? Ellen is the first to admit that she can't possibly answer that question. And although she is a medical doctor, she isn't even certain what caused her own healing. "I *do* know that what I learned was to use whatever vision I have," she says. This philosophy, together with her adherence to the eye exercise program, has enabled Ellen to see better than she has in many years.

Another alternative therapy system is "Integrated Visual Healing." It was developed by Grace Halloran, a woman whose own vision recovery is the result, she believes, of combining, in a very specific way, a number of alternative therapies. In addition to yoga, acupressure, nutrition, massage, and microcurrent stimulation, all designed to increase blood circulation in the retina, Halloran uses color therapy. This is a vibrational massage technique whereby specific hues are combined with specific light sources in front of the eye. The technique is thought to stimulate retinal cell activity and is designed to assist those whose ARMD has compromised their ability to differentiate color.

Some programs allege that deep-tissue massage, biofeedback, positive visualization, and a variety of nutritional supplements can act together to improve a patient's vision. From a medical perspective, scientific proof remains elusive. But this is not to say that well-informed patients, who can afford what often are expensive programs of this nature, should not participate. Most alternative therapists, many of whom have advanced academic degrees and/or some form of medical training, prefer the use of the term *adjunctive* or *complementary* therapies. Very few of them with established followings and satisfied clients would suggest that conventional medical advice and treatments ought to be ignored or eliminated. Instead they suggest that some or all of the less traditional Western therapies can prove very helpful when used in conjunction with standard medical programs or in situations where traditional medicine has few effective options to offer.

MEDITATION

Meditation, like yoga, is a practice that has come to us from other traditions and civilizations. Widely recommended for those whose lives are overloaded with obligations and activities, it is a way to regain a sense of control by taking two twenty-minute breaks per day. Although it requires practice to concentrate on your own breathing, and to release all other conflicting thoughts, many longtime practitioners of this discipline swear that it is the most mellowing and relaxing activity in their lives. Meditation classes, like yoga classes, are often given at community centers and YMCAs. You can also find a myriad of books on these practices, which are easy to master without individual instruction.

There are a number of holistic health practitioners who encourage their clients to embrace meditation or other forms of stress management, believing that the results will benefit eyesight specifically. Their view is not that meditation is a prescription that should be taken regularly like medication, but rather that less stress leads to a healthier body, and that a healthier body results in better eyesight.

HOMEOPATHY

Homeopathy is a scientific method of therapy based on the principle that the body's own healing process can be stimulated in order to facilitate its own cure. The founder of this treatment program was Samuel Hahnemann, a German physician who practiced at the turn of the eighteenth century. Homeopathy is not particularly well known in the United States, but it is widely practiced in other parts of the world, including Europe and India.

Homeopaths do not perform surgery. They prescribe

remedies, often very dilute herbal tinctures, in unique combinations based on an assessment of the patient's mental, emotional, and physical condition. Thus ten different patients with macular degeneration might receive ten different prescriptions from their homeopath, each reflecting that individual's unique characteristics.

There are homeopaths in most areas of the United States (though only three states—Arizona, Connecticut, and Nevada—offer a state licensing protocol), and the National Center for Homeopathy in Virginia maintains a directory for referrals. While few homeopaths would describe themselves as "retinal" or "macular degeneration specialists," one who has had a great deal of experience with treating eyes is Dr. Ed Kondrot of Pittsburgh, Pennsylvania. He is a licensed ophthalmologist who practiced conventional medicine for ten years before coming to the conclusion that "treating" his patients, particularly those with ARMD, was not the same as "curing" them. His study of homeopathy was an effort to move closer to that goal. During his nineteen years of practice as an ophthalmologist, he has seen hundreds of patients with ARMD. Not all are open to an "unconventional" homeopathic treatment program, but most of those who have embraced homeopathic remedies have generally been pleased with the results of their treatment.

Dr. Kondrot also uses microcurrent stimulation in his practice. After studying the results of sixty patients with dry ARMD on whom he used the treatment, 70 percent experienced an improvement of two or more lines on the eye chart. This improvement might be due to the microcurrent stimulating the transport mechanism for drusen material removal, but Dr. Kondrot does not know the exact mechanism responsible for it. He has been impressed, however, with the consistency of improvement in patients treated with microcurrent stimulation. He notes that one disadvantage is the need to keep reapplying the treatments.

Another therapy that Dr. Kondrot uses for ARMD patients is chelation therapy, whereby an antioxidant is introduced intravenously to precipitate out heavy metals and calcium from the blood. Calcium is one of the components of some types of drusen. This therapy is approved by the FDA, but only for use in vascular disease. Kondrot believes its use is best restricted to ARMD patients who also have atherosclerotic problems.

AEROBIC EXERCISE

I am often asked by physically active ARMD patients whether aerobic exercise such as running or tennis is harmful, or even causal, in the advancement of ARMD. As far as we know today, there is absolutely no evidence that strenuous aerobic exercise negatively affects ordinary age-related macular degeneration. While exercise of this nature does increase the rate at which blood flows through the circulatory system, this is not damaging to the macula—not even in patients who suffer from wet ARMD. Indeed, increased circulation is beneficial to overall health. If you have had laser surgery within two weeks, however, you should consult your ophthalmologist before resuming any type of exercise.

As a therapy for macular degeneration, there certainly are no data indicating that aerobic exercise is helpful in any way. Zealots, however, especially avid runners like my coauthor, Joan Snyder, believe that they are well when they are exercising strenuously every day, and less well when they're not. "I used to believe that I saw better after an eight- or ten-mile race than at any other time," Joan says, though even she, when pressed on the subject, admits that what she really felt after a long, hard run was the satisfaction of being strong enough and determined enough to complete it. She felt healthy, capable, and sure of herself, and these feelings are obviously the foundations of well-being. They are also, she adds, the perfect antidote for the psychological malaise that accompanies ARMD. Very few strenuous exercises require perfect sight, so for those to whom aerobic exercise is essential, macular degeneration is no impediment at all.

9

Promising Medical Research Initiatives

Because so many millions of people suffer from ARMD, and because the disease is affecting an ever-larger proportion of the U.S. population, there are many different treatment initiatives being pursued in diversified areas of health care. As a medical researcher, I am always most impressed by methodologies that have been rigorously tested and can be scientifically substantiated. But I am also sympathetic to the urgency many patients feel, and to their willingness to try almost anything to improve their failing sight.

While the standards of "proof" may be higher in the medical community than in the general patient population, I do not feel compelled to dissuade patients from trying "unproven" treatments except in three situations:

- If there may actually exist a health risk in experimenting with an unproven "cure."
- If, after asking questions and reading the materials

presented, you suspect you're being misled from a medical standpoint and you're needlessly depleting your financial resources.

- If scientific rigor is insufficient to really measure the results with accuracy, that is, the setting is not a bona fide clinical trial at an academic center but rather an experiment in an uncontrolled program.

When agents are tested in a clinical trial, there is a high level of quality control and consistency. Your results will be evaluated carefully, and it can be determined whether you are improving more dramatically than you might otherwise, had you not received any treatment. Additionally, the results of your experience will be properly cataloged so that the tested treatment can be made as effective as possible for others in need of similar therapies. In the context of an FDA-approved trial, not only are the intended results rigorously cataloged, side effects are recorded as well, even those that might not be instantly recognizable to a patient. Both your health and safety are protected, as well as those of future patients.

A list of clinical eye trials sponsored by the National Institutes of Health (NIH) can be found at the following Web site: http://www.nei.nih.gov/neitrials_script/ clin-alpha.asp.

SURGICAL PROCEDURES

Submacular Surgery

Over the last decade our surgical procedures have become increasingly sophisticated, and the tools used to

The Genetic Puzzle and Codes
That Might Crack It

There is considerable reason to speculate that a genetic basis exists for many diseases. ARMD is probably no exception. But even a scientifically well-grounded hunch cannot advance treatment or prevention until the specific genes implicated in the disease have been identified. Although specific genetic abnormalities have not yet been isolated for ARMD, genetic abnormalities have been found in diseases related to ARMD.

In Stargardt's disease there are drusen similar to those in ARMD. However, Stargardt's differs from ARMD in that it begins at a younger age and does not progress to blood vessel growth as commonly. Recently, Dr. Rando Allikmets at the NIH discovered that genetic abnormalities in the ABCR gene (also known as the photoreceptor rim protein) were a potential cause of Stargardt's disease. Some related genetic abnormalities were found in a number of patients with ARMD, but this finding has been contested by the scientific community because these abnormalities are thought by many to be present on a random basis and not actually causal in the development of ARMD.

Another disease known as Sorsby's dystrophy has some features similar to ARMD, such as the growth of new blood vessels under the retina. Mutations have been found in a gene known as TIMP-3 in patients with Sorsby's, a finding that is particularly intriguing.

A normal TIMP-3 gene inhibits blood vessel growth, so damage in this gene could potentially be responsible for the growth of blood vessels in Sorsby's dystrophy. Mutations in the TIMP-3 gene have not been found in patients with ARMD to date, but the finding is still a breakthrough for researchers in the field.

Identification of the mutant gene in a disease so closely related to ARMD has opened a very important window onto new information for researchers endeavoring to understand the genetic complexity of macular diseases. The next important task for medical research is to identify the way in which these particular genes act when causing disease. As in all serious detective work, even where the culprit is suspected, proof is essential. Isolating gene functions, both in their proper working form and in some deranged form that can cause disease, requires years of meticulous effort.

When this research is complete, it may be possible to transplant new genetic material to a diseased eye. DNA could literally be injected into the retina, with the expectation that the healthy genes within it would displace the mutant genes that had caused the patient's macula to deteriorate. The technology to successfully integrate new genes into the retina is not entirely proven, but neither is it merely wishful thinking. Many scientists believe that within the next five years, gene therapy for a variety of medical diseases will be as commonplace as heart bypass surgery is today for blocked arteries.

accomplish these techniques, equally advanced. Accordingly, ophthalmologists and retinal specialists in particular have sought new techniques to surgically remove the new blood vessels in the eye and the blood that remains from CNV. By making a hole in the side of the retina and sliding an instrument under the macula, it is possible to remove the CNV. Results from these procedures, however, have been mixed to date. We still lack sufficient information to tell us why the blood vessels regrow and continue to bleed, causing additional damage even after retinal surgery. Consequently, this invasive procedure, which cannot be repeated on a continuing basis for fear of damaging the eye more seriously than would the disease itself, will be most effective when our understanding of ARMD is further advanced.

Patients who have had submacular surgery generally had previously experienced a severe or total loss of vision in one eye and had reason to believe that the second eye would be similarly affected. Consider the case of Tim Jackson, who says that he had lost virtually all the vision in his left eye and had no problem with the right until one evening a year and a half later. "At 7:00 P.M. I was driving on a Denver interstate with no problems," he recalls. "At bedtime, I rubbed my eye and saw it hemorrhage, just like a dam breaking. In five seconds, I was far beyond legally blind." Tim had submacular surgery a few months later and now says, "I am grateful every day for what it did for my right eye. I regained some central sight, and it did wonders for the peripheral vision."

RPE Transplantation

An experimental surgical procedure known as RPE transplantation has been tried in a small group of patients. This technique involves the implantation of healthy human cells harvested from deceased donors into the diseased eye. Some researchers are experimenting with implantation of retinal pigment epithelial (RPE) cells from a patient's "good" eye into the "bad." The hope is that the RPE cells, the layer of cells that provides nourishment to the light-sensing cells in the eye, will be effectively rejuvenated by healthy tissue.

This procedure is being developed for use in conjunction with subretinal surgery. In a few experimental cases, the surgery was successful in replacing damaged RPE cells. But in other experiments, the new cells were rejected by the patient's immune system, so that no beneficial effect was achieved. Current research efforts are focused on reducing immune rejection and enhancing the survival and proliferation of the transplanted RPE cells.

Macular Translocation

In this experimental technique, the neurosensory portion of the macula is delicately moved to a slightly different location within the eye. To be effective at all, this procedure must be undertaken before macular deterioration has irretrievably damaged the fovea. The technique has been used so infrequently that we are not yet able to determine with certainty the opportunity that might be presented from this work.

After this surgery, the vision of some patients improved, but it had a distinct "tilt." Slightly skewed vision can often be improved over time, but it rarely disappears altogether. This condition might be considered only a minor disadvantage if the loss of central vision were the only other alternative faced by the patient, but the surgery itself has not been perfected, and many complications besides tilted vision have resulted where it has been tried. At this writing, experiments in the hands of qualified surgeons continue, and a clinical trial is being directed by Dr. Eugene De Juan in Baltimore.

Retinal Prosthesis

Also on the horizon is the creation and surgical implantation of a retinal prosthesis—in effect, an artificial retina. Inspired by promising initiatives with the cochlear prosthesis for the deaf (the "artificial ear"), scientists have begun experimenting with a "computer-chip" retina. For the device to work properly, the optic nerve must remain in healthy working order, which fortunately is the case with many ARMD patients (and just as many patients suffering from other eye diseases). Consequently, for those with advanced and very debilitating wet ARMD, a new lease on sighted life may be possible in the future from a retinal prosthesis.

RADIATION THERAPY

Another experimental course of treatment for CNV is gamma radiation therapy. There is moderate scientific data suggesting that this therapy might arrest the leakage of blood vessels. Protons are another very specific, highly focused form of radiation therapy most commonly used to treat melanoma. Approximately 1,000 cases have been reported in which radiation therapy was used on patients with both wet ARMD and PED. Some of the treated patients noticed an improvement in their sight, and some of their doctors reported less deterioration of vision than might otherwise have been expected, but the scientific rigor needed to verify these conclusions from a medical viewpoint has not yet been applied. In fact, recent data from a large European study of radiation for CNV found no difference between treated patients and the control group of patients. U.S. studies are still pending.

Radiation therapy is very similar to that used on tumors or other unwanted growths. It involves a highly focused beam of electromagnetic energy, that can kill tissue and theoretically destroy a troublesome blood vessel. It may leave behind a scar over the blood vessel, which could damage some vision, but the patient's overall ability to see may be generally improved. Radiation therapy does not seem to cause the immediate decline in visual acuity that is so often associated with laser therapy.

Radiation on human beings is always undertaken with extreme caution because the impact on dividing cells can be toxic. Radiation therapy for CNV may have permanent side effects, such as radiation retinopathy, which results in retinal damage and new vessel growth on the surface of the retina. Complex computer imaging is required to position both patient and instrumentation for precision application. Effective treatment of a minuscule blood vessel in the eye with radiation requires meticulous planning, highly sophisticated techniques, and, not incidentally, an enormous expense. This therapy is being investigated aggressively as a possible treatment for patients with wet ARMD, particularly because it appears to result in less severe vision loss than that experienced by patients treated with lasers.

STEROID INJECTIONS

In Australia trials are now being conducted to evaluate the promise of steroids, specifically triamcinolone, which is directly injected into the eye. The purpose of the treatment is not to eliminate the blood vessels but to reduce the leakage of fluid from them and hence the patient's experience of visual distortion. Steroid experiments previously focused on drops as a delivery system, which proved ineffective because the steroid could not reach the retina. Injections around the eye were similarly ineffective, but the current delivery system appears more promising. At the current time, there are no U.S. trials under way using this particular therapy, though medical researchers are following the Australian experiments with careful attention to their results. Similar trials are planned for the United States.

PART THREE

≈≈

Coping with
Age-Related
Macular Degeneration

10

~

Don't Give in to the Prognosis

The very term *macular degeneration* suggests a process of change over time. Negative change is clearly implied as your eyesight degenerates. Some ARMD patients say they would rather have a more serious illness that was static, where the primary psychological requirement is acceptance, and the fear of being worse tomorrow is removed. But in truth, virtually all disease is potentially degenerative, though most don't have such a malevolent descriptor as part of their name. Often it is not so much the notion of progressive deterioration that concerns patients, but rather the absence of any predictability about the timing of the progression. This randomness instills a sense of being out of control.

Patients may feel somewhat better if they always keep in mind the following three points:

1. Of the population diagnosed with ARMD, only 10 percent will experience deterioration to late-stage

ARMD with choroidal neovascularization. So the macula may degenerate over time—*but not necessarily.* ARMD is a diagnosis, not an immutable sentence. Some patients do, in fact, experience improvement in their vision from time to time, and many never experience noticeable vision degeneration at all.

2. Even if the macula does continue to degenerate, most patients have just a mild vision loss. Only a very small proportion develop severe visual impairment.

3. Patients are not blind, even if they fit the legal definition, and they will not become totally blind from ARMD.

The prognosis for this disease is comparatively straightforward. We know that eyesight generally deteriorates over time, and that glasses are normally required to improve distance or reading capability in the vast majority of older adults. However, there are rare cases where the symptoms of age-related macular degeneration do, in fact, reverse themselves. Even with wet ARMD, improvement is possible. In a study of patients with diminished vision from subfoveal, subretinal hemorrhage—an abnormal bleeding vessel right under the crucial fovea where laser treatment is not recommended—21 percent of the subjects had improved vision of three or more lines on the eye chart three years after the bleeding episode.* Vision changes may be fleeting, or they may be prolonged. The long-term

*R. L. Avery et al., *Retina* 16, no. 3 (1996):183–89.

trend may be downward, but there may well be intervals of both gradual and dramatic improvement. And there may very likely be prolonged stability.

Although there are limited treatments available at the moment and only working theories about how to halt the progression of the disease, we in the medical research community are optimistic about the possibility of a cure in the near future. In the meanwhile, there are many things that patients with ARMD can do to lead active, fulfilling lives.

ACTIVE VERSUS PASSIVE REACTIONS

Mary Laneer is a nurse in Chicago. She has worked for many years with a pain management clinic that helps patients cope with relentless, incurable pain. When she was diagnosed with late-stage wet ARMD, Mary made only one change in her life: She determined to accept the reality of her condition. Acceptance is easy to talk about and far more difficult to achieve, but Mary is well aware of the physical destruction that results from fighting the insurmountable difficulties in life. She has seen firsthand the impact of stress-related symptoms—symptoms unrelated to a specified disease, symptoms unrelated to localized pain—when patients internalize anger and fight the inevitable.

Acceptance is not passive; it is, in fact, an active choice that allows you to stare an ugly reality in the face and move on. Mary is well aware that her vision may gradually diminish; although she has made no tangible plans to change her life, she relies a bit more on others for assistance and doesn't much worry that her reputation as wholly self-reliant might need to be revised at some point. She is neither happy nor sad that she has ARMD. She is merely accepting.

Todd Freeman is a mechanical engineer whose defining belief in life is that he can fix anything—a belief supported by five decades of home improvements and professional achievements. His ARMD is still in its early stages, and in fact his symptoms of poor vision in dim light and his decreased sensitivity to color contrast have not changed in over three years. But if they do, he will be ready.

He has read every book on the subject of ARMD, knows every Web site dedicated to vision problems, and has a wide range of magnifiers in boxes, ready for use when he needs them. He has rewired his house to provide for bright lighting virtually everywhere and has enough floodlights in his garden to make it resemble a prison yard at night. Todd is more than prepared for the worst. He's prepared for anything. His view is that planning and preparation make him feel safe; that being in control, even if his eyesight is out of control, makes him believe that he still has choices left, choices which will make his life rewarding and productive.

Mary and Todd may represent extremes, but they both illustrate the point that a strong psychological defense suited to one's one personality is as important in coping with ARMD as a coherent medical strategy. Ideally, one can take a bit of each example and use it to one's advantage. Acceptance is a prerequisite for coping calmly and effectively with anything, especially with disease. But an active, vigorous program to take charge of your life, in the face of illness, is equally desirable.

Whether or not modern medicine can deliver reliable treatments for a disease, patients usually have the potential to improve their condition. In the case of ARMD, science is slow in delivering on its promise, but you must not assume then that you, as a patient, have no role to play. On the contrary, you are in charge of your reactions. The more positive they are, within the context of your own personality and lifestyle, the less impact the disease will have, regardless of your specific symptoms.

THREE BASIC ACTIONS

One of the common mantras used by those dealing with ARMD is "Move it over, light it up, make it bigger." Taking these three actions will help you maximize your vision.

Move It Over

When some or all of your central vision is impaired, the way to compensate is to move the object you want to see to the side. This enables you to use your peripheral vision, the nonmacular part of your retina, to see. Move your magazine to each side, and you'll get a sharper image of the photograph on the page. Hold your bridge cards slightly to the left or right of the center of your vision; both the suit and the number should come into clearer focus.

There are immovable objects in the world, as we all know, so when a mountain can't be moved, you will need to turn your head. Begin to develop a slightly off-center way of looking, moving your eyes to both sides of the object you want to examine. The image will not be as clear or as steady as when you were able to see it well face-on, but it will not be altogether absent. With practice, you will still be able to see the faces on Mt. Rushmore, the Christmas tree at Rockefeller Center, and the smile on your new grandchild's face.

Light It Up

Bright light will help enormously, especially for early-stage ARMD patients. Halogen lights are particularly useful for close work, and direct lighting over any reading material is essential. If you have trouble reading the program in the concert hall, the menu in a restaurant, or the book at prayer, take along a miniature flashlight. The external environment is not always easy to improve, but in your home, you can control the type and the amount of light, which should enable you to see much better. For more tips on lighting, see the discussion in chapter 11.

Make It Bigger

Large-print books and newspapers can be purchased in bookstores and are also available in libraries. If you have a small blind spot in your vision, large print may fall outside the blind spot and thus be easier to read. If you have a large blind spot, large print may not fill in the blanks, but your brain will react more quickly to easily readable letters and fill in the missing bits with less effort. AARP, the American Association of Retired Persons, sometimes uses strong, bold black print on its credit card statements and many of its circulars. Some materials are printed in white letters on a dark background, a format that certain ARMD patients find helpful in eliminating glare. This organization realizes that ARMD has affected much of its membership, and that big, bold print is much easier for those individuals to read.

Magnifiers are also helpful for reading and other close work. We'll examine magnification in more detail in chapter 11.

SEEING IN THE DARK

Contrast is a necessary component of vision. The higher the contrast, the easier it is to recognize an object. You will see poorly in dark rooms or outdoors at night because the decreased contrast will diminish your overall visual acuity. The extent of these limitations varies widely in ARMD patients, but it is one of the consequences of the disease that patients find most troublesome. They also find it dangerous, because many entrance halls in public spaces, like restaurants, are poorly lit. Entering a dark space from a brightly lit parking lot can cause many people to trip and fall, even those with perfect sight.

Driving at night also becomes problematic, especially on back roads and country lanes. Some patients find that amber-tinted lenses are helpful in heightening contrast and reducing the glare of oncoming headlights; others find that gold antireflective coatings on their eyeglasses are superior, especially if they are very sensitive to bright light. But if your visual limitations make it difficult for you to drive at night, it is pointless to "try to drive." You endanger your own life and the lives of others as well. Your participation in many activities will not be limited by your sight impairment; in these cases, seeing less well is annoying but doesn't pose any risks. Driving is not one of those activities, however.

GETTING BY IN SOCIAL SITUATIONS

Impaired vision is a serious problem. As anyone with ARMD knows, there are many major compromises to be made in life if the disease has progressed to the point where you are really dependent upon others for assistance. What is often overlooked, however, is the fact that it is not the monumental moments but the mundane things in daily life that can often be the most troublesome. Consider, for example, the act of eating. One ARMD patient tried to eat peanuts from a bowl at a cocktail party, but those nuts that looked so desirable turned out to be merely the pattern on an ashtray.

When the fear of committing a faux pas—like attempted ashtray consumption—threatens to restrain your socializing, it is important to remember that there are a few techniques that can be used to ease difficult situations. If you socialize with a partner or the same group of friends regularly, rely on them to provide unobtrusive assistance. More stress results from pretending you have perfect vision than from simply recognizing your limitations.

If you're comfortable discussing your vision with your host or hostess, be direct; ask what's being served when you accept an invitation, and think about any difficulties you might encounter at the dinner table. It will keep you from endeavoring to peel a shrimp that turns out to be a steak bone, as author Henry Grunwald recalled doing once in *Twilight*. Don't serve yourself or others unless you are confident you can move peas from a serving bowl to a plate without any runaways. Learn to accept that when help is offered, the offer is almost always sincere; and when help isn't offered, most people are pleased to be asked.

In *Twilight*, Grunwald describes his experience with age-related macular degeneration, recounting many poignant moments of confusion, some hilarious, such as when he tried valiantly to distinguish the gender symbols on the rest-room doors in a restaurant. When, in the course of an average day, you realize that you're wearing a sweater inside out, you spill soda all over your desk by setting the can down on thin air, and you are unable to distinguish between coins and tokens when you get to the bus, it's time to reassess your approach. These are not the results of poor vision or of ARMD per se; they are the consequences of poor planning or pride. ARMD will mean slowing your life down and relying more on others—friends and strangers alike.

ADAPTIVE BEHAVIORS

Obviously you will face limitations with ARMD, and the first order of the day is to keep your expectations of yourself within reasonable bounds. This may mean cutting back. It may mean that you can no longer complete the Sunday morning crossword puzzle. But there may be a substitution that will give you equal pleasure.

Finding New Hobbies

Activity	Substitute Found
Hand sewing	Rug hooking Rather than strain to see minute stitches, Margaret uses a huge latch, thick yarn, and makes beautiful throw rugs for Christmas gifts.
Reading	Listening to recorded books Phil now listens to books read by professional readers and has organized a book club with neighbors to discuss the books its members either read or hear.
Writing letters	Long, leisurely phone conversations Phone calls cost a bit more but provide more intimacy.
Woodworking	Nature hikes Matt can no longer see well enough to work safely around power tools. What he always loved best about woodworking was the smell of the lumber, which he now recollects in every pleasurable smell of the woods.
Sailing	Canoeing Kathy felt she couldn't sail compet-

itively any longer because she couldn't see as well as her other crewmates. Her love of the water turned her to canoeing, where visual acuity is less urgent.

Tennis	Swimming When Day-Glo balls still can't be seen well enough to return a fast serve, take up a sport like swimming that requires different skills.
Gardening	Dog obedience training Sometimes a total shift is most rewarding; one that is interactive with a pet can be particularly satisfying (and helpful if you have a badly behaved dog).
Stamp collecting	Regular museum visits Randy found that he could see many of the larger exhibits well and enjoyed the interactive ones particularly.
Flying	Hot-air-balloon rides Tim had been a pilot all his life, but blurry controls grounded him. Now he treats himself to hot-air balloon rides with a copilot who takes care of the details while Tim enjoys the sense of flying free.

Consider playing one of the interactive computer games where you can increase the type to virtually any size letters you like, or listening to books on tape, or engaging in another quiet pastime. The important point is to replace the lost activity with another that provides the same quality of enjoyment but does not depend upon perfect eyesight.

Over the years, my patients have told me about the many adaptations they've made in their activities. I am awestruck by the creativity of their solutions to what often appear to be insurmountable difficulties. The accompanying box presents nine activities that my patients have had to give up and nine others that have served as satisfactory replacements.

To replace a longtime hobby with a new activity, one needs to be flexible and willing to make changes. Clinging to past behaviors is a defensive strategy that comes naturally to all of us. But if you can adjust your life by finding new pleasures and reveling in them, what is lost to you will not seem as significant. In fact, some of my patients have used their ARMD diagnosis as an opportunity to make changes in other areas of their lives as well.

Leslie Aames, for example, has been on multiple medications for many years. She has allergy pills, blood pressure pills, and a variety of mild pain medications for the dental work she has endured. Her age-related macular degeneration made her do what her friends and family had been telling her to do for years: throw out all old medications, and clearly identify those that remain. Because Leslie is unable to read the fine print on the bottles, even with the magnifier she now keeps in the bathroom, she devised a clever system for identifying her medications.

In her desk drawer, typed in a very large, bold font, is a chart of codes for the medications. (She keeps it for reference, but her memory is excellent and she rarely needs to use it.) The codes for her regular medications are as follows: A strip of Velcro on the bottle identifies allergy pills; rubber bands around the bottle mean blood pressure medication; and an aluminum foil wrap covers the bottle containing calcium supplements. These textures are obvious to Leslie the minute she picks up the bottles. Her grandson spray-painted with wild metallic colors the tops of a couple of other medications she uses less regularly. The colors are easy for her to see, and her large-print chart in the drawer also includes the color codes for these medications.

Those who live alone find ARMD more debilitating than those who live with others willing to offer assistance. Everything, from turning the oven dial to a designated temperature to reading instructions on a can of ant poison, requires some central vision, and the more of it you lose, the less capable you feel yourself becoming. It's true that dials can be marked with touch-sensitive tape at certain intervals, and that the Poison Control Center can tell you over the phone all you need to know about spraying in the kitchen. But if you are living alone and have ARMD, sooner or later you are going to conclude that a helpful hand is required.

Fred Steamer has lived alone since his wife died. His only daughter and her family live 2,000 miles away. He considered moving across the country to be with them, but he is attached to his own community and enjoys his independence in the home he has lived in for forty years. Fred's ARMD is advanced enough that cooking for himself is difficult, driving, all but impossible, and living alone, less satisfying. The thought of having a stranger come in to "treat me like an invalid" was appalling, as was the notion of moving to an assisted living facility. It was his closest friend's son, a professor at a nearby college, who suggested that what Fred needed was an almost invisible roommate—one who would understand and respect Fred's desire for independence, but who would be available for general help and assistance at certain times of the day. A note posted on the student bulletin board immediately produced a solution.

Now living harmoniously near the village of Manchester, Vermont, are a stubborn old gentleman with limited sight and a feisty young college senior who is thrilled with his comfortable surroundings. In exchange for free room and board, Sam cooks better meals than Fred has eaten in years and looks after chores that he describes as needing "young eyes." Fred is the first to admit that asking for help was not easy for him, and that his "image" was almost more important than his sight in some ways. Today, his self-esteem is still intact, and his life is infinitely more comfortable thanks to this unconventional solution to the need for "assistive eyes."

I have seen many patients with age-related macular degeneration over the years. Some cope well, even brilliantly. Others, once diagnosed, never enjoy themselves fully ever again. Although optimism cannot be prescribed, and there is no pill that will encourage those who have difficulty adjusting to the diagnosis, I hope the stories in this chapter will inspire you to stay active and get the most out of life.

11

✐

Low-Vision Support Tools

No matter what type or what stage of ARMD you are dealing with, you can use a number of vision devices that will make daily living a good deal more manageable. Low-vision support devices are still in their early stages of development. Many are clumsy, few are especially portable, but they are helpful aids that will vastly improve your vision—provided you use them correctly.

Your goal should be to adopt realistic expectations about the future, based on a professional rehabilitator's evaluation, and to focus on task-specific objectives. Certainly it is desirable to "see better" in general, but it is much more useful to identify specific activities or specific situations that for you, individually, are especially significant. Working on these priorities first, your world will brighten immeasurably. A low-vision rehabilitator can give you considerable advice on coping with common problems found in the house or at work, but that expert will be much more helpful to you if you prioritize the activities or situations that tend to be recurrent problems in your life.

REFRACTIVE CORRECTION

The first line of defense in maximizing your vision is a pair of glasses that are suited to your needs. Spectacles will correct whatever can be corrected by refraction. If you have relatively good vision in one eye but are myopic (nearsighted) or hyperopic (farsighted), that particular vision deficiency can be corrected. It is not possible to correct the damage of ARMD with glasses, nor even to compensate with glasses, but you still can expect some improvement with spectacles or contact lenses that address your other visual needs.

Don't expect that you can select glasses from a supermarket shelf and find the optimal correction. Proper refraction for low-vision patients requires meticulous effort, and you should see a low-vision specialist who is willing and able to spend the necessary time to produce the right glasses for you. This specialist can also give you information on how best to become accustomed to new glasses, and how to maximize your vision while wearing them. There are optometrists and opticians who specialize in working with low-vision patients, and many of these professionals have assistive-device trainers working in their offices.

For patients with more serious visual handicaps, glasses that incorporate both a corrective feature and a properly balanced degree of magnification may be particularly helpful. These glasses greatly magnify the material being read, if it is held close enough. Some patients find that their field of vision is so limited that it is distracting. Depending upon the necessary correction and degree of magnification, often it is only possible to see a few words at a time. This can make reading quite tiresome, but most patients with severe vision loss appreciate being able to read at least the "small essentials"—like directions on bottles or "fine print" labels that are always, infuriatingly, illegible to virtually all eyes over forty.

Special prescriptions can also be obtained for filters or coatings that block out certain types of light. For example, there are gold-colored coatings that can be helpful in reducing glare outdoors, and plum-colored coatings that are effective indoors. Not all patients find these special colors helpful, but many do, and a low-vision specialist will often allow you to try out specialized glasses, recognizing that their effectiveness is highly variable from patient to patient. If the glasses aren't helpful, you may be able to return them.

Photophobia, the medical term for extreme light sensitivity, which some patients with retinal problems experience, sounds like a minor problem easily addressed with a pair of very dark sunglasses, but this is an effective correction only for people with normal eyesight. Some patients actually report intensely unpleasant glare from sunlight bouncing off their cheeks on very bright days. TV viewing for these people is impossible because of constant variations in light on the screen, and prolonged computer use can be agonizing. "I live like a mole or a bat," one patient told me. "I try to go out only late in the afternoon or early in the evening, though that doesn't help much if I have to go to a store that has fluorescent lights."

Photophobia can sometimes be addressed by use of several different pairs of glasses for different light conditions, including amber and dark green tints. Ski goggles also can help, especially those that eliminate light from the top, bottom, and sides. Some can even be custom-ground to corrective specifications, and tinted to a customized degree of color, with darker tint, for example, on the side shields.

ILLUMINATION

The single most effective support tool, particularly for reading or other close work, is a proper lamp. One of the best is referred to as an "architect's lamp"; it has a minimum of 100 watts of incandescent illumination. The lamp is most effective when placed approximately eight inches from the reading material. Glare is minimized by keeping the light source positioned to the side but between you and your reading material. Halogen and fluorescent lighting also provide bright light, but often the glare is excessive, actually compounding vision difficulties for ARMD patients. A 150-watt incandescent light provides warm, gentle tone, and full-spectrum, or chromalux, bulbs can be used to filter out yellow rays that sometimes dull perception of color or detail.

MAGNIFICATION AND OTHER LOW-VISION TOOLS

In general, there are three kinds of magnification: relative distance magnification, relative size magnification, and angular magnification. The first allows objects that are at a distance to look bigger when brought closer;

when, for example, you are trying to thread a needle, this type of magnification is crucial. Relative size magnification is what virtually everyone over forty needs to read the telephone directory. Angular magnification is used in binoculars and telescopes. All three kinds of magnification are incorporated in different types of assistive devices for the visually impaired. A low-vision expert can explain the purpose and procedure for using each.

Magnifying lamps are also helpful for hobbies and other close work. Magnifiers with built-in lighting are available on flexible arms to be attached to a table, or as standing units to swing in front of a chair or over a table. While they take a bit of getting used to, they are generally very helpful to patients with atrophic or early-stage ARMD. Handheld magnifiers, many of which include battery-operated lights, are immensely useful for reading maps, price tags, and menus.

Other low-vision tools that provide help to ARMD patients include:

- Closed-circuit-TV reading devices. A small, hand-held "mouse" slides across a map or a printed page, for example, and the image is projected onto either a TV or a computer screen. Magnification is variable.
- "Talking" clock-radios, VCRs, wristwatches, bathroom scales, and compasses that audibly announce the information that would otherwise be read.
- Large-button phones, remote-control devices, and indoor/outdoor thermometers.
- Signature guides and check-writing templates to guide your hand to the proper lines.

• Specialized high-intensity flashlights, some of which are feather light, have flexible necks, and, as battery-operated units, can be clipped onto a cap.

These are just a few of the many devices that have been designed to assist those with low vision. For a listing of companies and organizations offering these and other useful products or services, see the "Resources" section.

YOUR HOME ENVIRONMENT

If you have ARMD, it is important to make your own environment as responsive to that condition as possible. Accidents are frequently the result of not being able to see well, and for elders particularly, falls can cause serious injuries.

Around the House

• For security, an intercom can be installed at the front door, enabling visitors to identify themselves even if they can't be seen well.
• Wireless sensor lights can be easily installed in the entry area of the house so that they will always provide light, even if you leave when it is daylight and return after dark. An inexpensive alternative is to use an automatic night-light in the entry area.
• All walkways in the garden should be landscaped along the edge with plant material that provides a clear contrast to the color of the walkways.
• Paths should be well lit at night with solar or low-voltage lights, and outdoor stairs should be marked

on their edges with paint or a strip of tape in a contrasting color.

- Open patios or decks should be cleared of low tables or benches to provide clear space in the center, with furniture grouped around the outside perimeter.

Living Spaces

- It is easier to see furniture when its color contrasts with that of the floor or the carpet; edges of couches are more visible if they are piped with brightly colored cord.
- Sheer curtains and blinds will reduce glare if you are particularly sensitive to light.
- Install automatic lighting in closets, and arrange clothes by color groupings.
- Consider installing electrical outlets that are illuminated or whose color contrasts with the wall color.
- Eliminate or tape down all scatter rugs, and remove unused clutter from rooms.

Kitchen and Bathrooms

- Countertops should be painted, taped, or built with contrasting-color edges. Burners on the cooktop should provide some contrast; there are also halogen cooktops on which the burners turn bright red when hot.
- If dials are difficult to read, frequently used settings on the stove can be clearly marked with nail polish, as can all the "off" positions.
- Some microwaves have sensor reheat features, so that reading the numbers is less critical.

- Use chopping boards of different colors, so that light-colored foods can be chopped on a dark surface, and vice versa.
- Install waterproof lights in the shower and in the bathtub area.

12

〰

The Low-Vision Community

You are not alone. For anyone who suffers from age-related macular degeneration, it is often comforting to know that many millions of other people are in the same boat. Individually and together they have forged strategies and developed techniques that make their vision problems more manageable. Often, just sharing stories with others who completely empathize with your problem can be an uplifting experience.

This chapter discusses some of the organizations and Web sites that you may find particularly helpful. Additional organizations are listed in the "Resources" section.

NATIONAL SUPPORT GROUPS

The Macular Degeneration Foundation is a nonprofit foundation created by patients to help fight macular degeneration. Physicians who are part of the foundation help clarify medical information for their members. The foundation publishes a newsletter with up-to-date information on developments in the area of macular degeneration and maintains a useful and informative Web site. Contact:

Macular Degeneration Foundation
Tel.: (888) 633-3937
Web site: http://www.eyesight.org

On this site are reports of new research breakthroughs, links to other relevant sites, technical references, and descriptions of new initiatives. Because the site is maintained by a knowledgeable professional in the field of ocular medicine, it is a dependable source for evaluation of technical issues. The foundation also supports new research initiatives. I serve as a science adviser to the Macular Degeneration Foundation.

Another helpful resource is the Lighthouse International in your area. This nonprofit, nonaffiliated organization, formerly known as the Lighthouse for the Blind, is dedicated to assisting those with eyesight impairment of any nature, not just those who are blind. Contact:

Lighthouse International
Tel.: (800) 829-0500
Web site: http://www.lighthouse.org

This organization can help you find services nationwide, including support groups, recreation resources, and vision rehabilitation centers. It also has a catalog of products specifically suited to those with vision problems. The goal of Lighthouse International is to assist people with sight problems to live independently; its educational programs, special events, and research activities are particularly helpful to ARMD sufferers.

You can also find local support at your chapter of the American Association of Retired Persons (AARP). Contact the national headquarters for information:

AARP
Tel.: (800) 424-3410
Web site: http://www.aarp.org

An excellent source of information for elders is your Area Agency on Aging. The national umbrella organization in Washington, D.C., can provide you with a local number. Contact:

The Elder Locator
Tel.: (800) 677-1116
Web site: http://www.aoa.dhhs.gov/

This organization is prepared to answer many questions about the services available to elders in state and local offices. Many of these service bureaus can provide a local list of low-vision opticians, ophthalmologists, and optometrists. Though there are differences in various states, most states have a Bureau of Services for the Visually Impaired (BSVI) or a Sight Services for Independent Living. Both agencies typically offer counseling and training with low-vision devices. Sometimes the programs are organized under the state's department of vocational rehabilitation. A bit of searching through the listings for local government offices in your phone book will lead you to a wealth of publicly funded resources.

HELPFUL WEB SITES

One of the most direct ways to be in touch with other ARMD patients is through the Internet. If you have put off the idea of becoming cyber-connected, this is an opportunity to make progress on two fronts: You can learn a new skill while you gain information on your eye condition, chatting with others whose sight has been compromised or with friends and relatives of those who are learning to live with diminished sight.

While writing this book, my coauthor signed on to the MDList, a Web site with postings from those interested in ARMD, hoping to hear more about patients' major concerns and their strategies for coping. What she found was a group of enormously supportive individuals whose ages (early twenties to late eighties) and lifestyles (college student to space-program engineer) differ enormously, but all of whom have two things in common: macular degeneration and, more important, optimism. The Web address for MDList is:

http://members.aol.com/danlrob/MDpeople/
mdlist.html

Many MDList subscribers have been actively chatting with others for a long time, but new patients and new relatives of patients log on daily with questions, ideas, suggestions, and references. Each is welcomed by literally hundreds of new friends and individually by the guiding light of the MDList, Dan Roberts. There are few subjects in this book that have not been discussed in detail by many patients whose personal experiences are both instructive and inspirational. The same group has its own Internet bookstore, which carries many titles dealing with ARMD and similar vision problems.

My coauthor and I asked everyone on the MDList what had been, for each of them, the single most helpful thing in coping with ARMD or in helping a loved one cope with the disease. Their answers, broadly categorized, were as follows:

- *faith*, in its many varied forms, which led inevitably to a more positive attitude;
- *support systems*, composed of family, community groups, and, very frequently, the MDList community itself; and
- *technology*, including, most important, the computer.

Because ARMD has affected many who did not grow up using interactive technology, it is often difficult to think that the computer is a promising solution, since it presents, at the outset, a steep initial learning curve. This is particularly true to the extent that low vision is too often accompanied by low confidence, especially as vision worsens. But there are universities and community centers that provide computer training for senior citizens, and many specific programs through more specialized venues such as low-vision clinics.

The computer offers not only access to and friendship with many other ARMD patients, but technological solutions to some of the most serious losses in a patient's life, such as the ability to read. With a computer, one can buy products that scan books and read them back (Open Book Unbound), others that read aloud whatever is written on the screen (JAWS), and programs that focus on small parts of the screen with magnification (Zoomtext). A helpful site for the many resources dedicated to computer use by the blind is the following:

http://www.hicom.net/~oedipus/blist.html

Even though most of the information available is in the English language, translation help for many other languages can be found:

http:/www.babelfish.com

Most large public libraries and university libraries have reading rooms for the visually impaired. Often their equipment includes sophisticated computer workstations enhanced for low-vision and braille-dependent patrons. Even in smaller libraries there are often tape players and a selection of recorded books. Call your library to inquire about the special services and instruction offered, and for information on the easiest physical access to the building.

Another useful source for book lovers is "Bookmania," a visual-impairment department operated in conjunction with Amazon Co., UK. Their Web site address is:

http://www.website1.freeserve.com.uk/index2.html

The site is in large print on easy-to-read background colors and designed for those who wish to order books online but have trouble reading the screen of most booksellers.

There is also a remarkably complete Web site designed by Elizabeth Hamilton, coordinator of services to patrons with print disabilities at the University Libraries, University of Cincinnati. Hamilton, who herself has low vision, trains patrons to use the Internet and the library's online databases. Her Web site offers resources for people with a variety of print disabilities, including "Windows Tips for Users with Low Vision," a guide you may download or print that is specifically designed for neophyte computer users. The Web addresses for the guide are:

http://w3.one.net/~hamlite/disab/wintip95.html
(for Windows 95)
http://w3.one/~hamilte/disab/wintip31.html
(for Windows 3.1)

There are tips on how to modify certain features to make reading easier, reduce glare, and enhance color. (For example, many new computer users find that changing the color settings to yellow print on a blue background screen gives them the most legible format.)

Even for those whose vision is not impaired, the guide is a very simple, compact explanation of the Windows operating system and helpful to those starting out on the computer, whether with this or later versions of Windows.

EPILOGUE

There is ample reason to believe that medicine and science will soon make breakthroughs in preventing and, we hope, curing ARMD in both its wet and dry manifestations. The rate of progress on the medical front is accelerating, and treatments for the disease will almost surely be improved, if not perfected, in the next several years.

But scientific breakthroughs require not only wisdom and mastery of technical details, but also funding to support millions of hours of necessary research. In this respect, ARMD, though it affects a large segment of our population, must compete with other diseases for a fair share of scarce financial resources.

If you have the funds and the desire to make a donation to one (or more) of the myriad efforts directed toward ARMD medical research, see the list of worthy organizations provided in the "Resources" section for suggestions in this regard.

A gift of equal import is the direct communication of your concerns about ARMD to those who make decisions on where research dollars are spent. Letters requesting that more funding be made available for research will alert funding authorities to the public's mounting concerns. It is, after all, the public will that ultimately determines how government resources are allocated. And that will is manifest in the cumulative impact of each individual who speaks up and asks that a cure for ARMD be found NOW!

GLOSSARY

ABCR gene: A gene recently found by medical researchers that may ultimately be significant in identifying the causes of, and possibly a cure for, a disease similar to ARMD known as Stargardt's.

Amsler Grid: A self-screening tool to identify possible vision problems.

Angiogenesis inhibition: A function that blocks blood vessel growth.

Angiogram: A medical test administered to examine the retina.

Carotenoids: Pigments found in plants that have the ability to absorb light.

Choroid: The bottom layer of blood vessels under the retina.

Choroidal neovascularization, or CNV: A technical term for abnormal blood vessel growth under the retina, a condition that leads to a diagnosis of wet ARMD.

Cones: Cells found in the photoreceptor layer of the retina that are used in conjunction with rods and that are primarily responsible for one's ability to see color and detail.

Cornea: A transparent membrane that sits on the outside of the eyeball.

Disciform scar: The end result of a blood vessel that has leaked, causing vision impairment. May cause a blind spot known as a *scotoma.*

Drusen: Waste material under the retina, the appearance of which may signify the possibility of current or future macular degeneration.

Fluorescein: A dye used in the administration of an angiogram test.

Fovea: The center point of the macula that provides detailed vision in a healthy eye.

Hyperopia: The technical term for someone who is commonly referred to as "farsighted."

Indocyanine green: A dye used as an alternative to fluorescein in the administration of an angiogram test.

Iris (sing.), Irides (pl.): The colored portion of the front of the eye that surrounds the pupil.

Laser: In the context of ocular medicine, a form of light that is sometimes applied in the treatment of age-related macular degeneration.

Lutein: A form of carotenoid found in fruits and vegetables that appears to be linked to ocular health.

Macula: The center portion of the retina, wherein one's central focusing ability is found.

Macular translocation: An experimental surgical procedure in which a portion of the macula is relocated within the eye.

Microcurrent stimulation: A procedure being tested to treat age-related macular degeneration using extremely low-voltage electrical stimulation.

Myopia: The technical term for the condition commonly referred to as nearsightedness.

Ophthalmologist: A medical doctor trained in diseases of the eye and qualified to perform corrective surgery.

Optician: A technician trained to produce and dispense corrective lenses.

Optometrist: A medical specialist who deals with the correction of vision problems but who is not trained to perform surgery.

Photocoagulation: A term for laser treatment sometimes applied to patients with ARMD, especially in its wet form.

Photodynamic therapy: A specific type of therapy, similar to laser, for treatment of age-related macular degeneration that may offer superior, post-therapeutic results.

Photoreceptors: Light-sensing cells located in the retina. Photoreceptors are made up of rods and cones.

Proton treatment: A type of radiation therapy.

Radiation therapy: The use of highly focused electromagnetic energy to destroy unwanted tissue or blood vessels.

Retina: The most important tissue layer in the eye, connected to the optic nerve.

Rods: Cells found in the photoreceptor layer of the retina that are used in conjunction with cones and that are primarily responsible for one's ability to see in the dark.

Sclera: The tissue layer on the outer portion of the eye that appears as the "white of the eye."

Submacular surgery: An experimental surgical procedure to remove a blood vessel.

**Transcutaneous electrical nerve stimulation (TENS)
unit:** A mechanical device used in microcurrent
stimulation.

Triamcinolone: A steroid being tested in Australian
clinical trials to determine its effectiveness in reducing bleeding from wet ARMD.

Zeaxanthin: A type of carotenoid found in fruits and
vegetables that appears to be associated with good
ocular health.

RESOURCES

Not-for-Profit Foundations and Associations

The following are dedicated to finding a cure for ARMD and to assisting those who are afflicted:

American Foundation for the Blind
11 Penn Plaza, Suite 300
New York, NY 10001
Tel.: (800) 232-5463
     (212) 502-7600
Web site: http://www.afb/org

Foundation Fighting Blindness
1401 Mt. Royal Avenue
Baltimore, MD 21217
Tel.: (800) 638-5551

Lighthouse International
111 East Fifty-ninth Street
New York, NY 10022
Tel.: (800) 829-0500
       (212) 821-9200
Web site: www.lighthouse.org

The Macula Foundation
519 East Seventy-second Street, Suite 203
New York, NY 10021
Tel.: (212) 605-3777

Macular Degeneration Foundation
P.O. Box 9752
San Jose, CA 95157
Tel.: (888) 633-3937
       (408) 260-1335
Fax: (408) 260-1330
Web site: http://www.eyesight.org

The National Association for Visually Handicapped
22 West Twenty-first Street
New York, NY 10010
Tel.: (212) 889-3141
Fax: (212) 727-2931
E-mail: staff@navh.org
Web site: http://www.navh.org

Other Organizations

American Academy of Ophthalmology
This nonprofit organization is the largest national
membership association of ophthalmologists in the

United States. It includes more than 90 percent of the practicing ophthalmologists in the United States, and more than 5,000 international members.

The academy maintains a Web site that can lead you to its member retinal specialists in any U.S. city, or you can call the academy for direct assistance.

MAILING ADDRESS
P.O. Box 7424
San Francisco, CA 94120
STREET ADDRESS FOR MAIL DELIVERY SERVICES
655 Beach Street
San Francisco, CA 94109
Tel.: (415) 561-8500
Fax: (415) 561-8575
Web site: http://www.eyenet.org

American Association of Naturopathic Physicians
601 Valley Street, Suite 105
Seattle, WA 98109
Tel.: (206) 298-0126
Fax: (206) 298-0129
Web site: http://www.naturopathic.org

Low-Vision Association of Ontario
This organization has a broader reach than the name implies. As a member, you are part of a "virtual" association on the Internet.
101-263 Russell Hill Road
Toronto, Ontario M4V 2TA
Web site: http://www.lowvision.on.ca

Where to Find Vision Aid Products (New and Used)

Access with Ease
1755 Johnson P.O. Box 1150
Chino Valley, AZ 86323
Tel.: (800) 531-9479 (orders)
      (520) 636-9469
Fax: (520) 636-0292

Allied Technologies of Virginia
4317 Heremleigh Lane
Mechanicsville, VA 23111
Tel.: (888) 781-0425
E-mail: AlliedVA@aol.com
Web site: http://www.LowVis.com

The Lighthouse Catalog
36-20 Northern Boulevard
Long Island City, NY 11101
Tel.: (800) 829-0500
E-mail: lighthousecatalog@lighthouse.org
Web site: http://www.lighthouse.org

LS&S Group
P.O. Box 673
Northbrook, IL 60065
Tel.: (800) 468-4789
Fax: (847) 498-1482
E-mail: LSSGRP@aol.com

Maxi-Aides Catalog
P.O. Box 3209
Farmington, NY 11735
Tel.: (800) 522-6294

Noir Medical Technologies
P.O. Box 159
6155 Pontiac Trail
South Lyon, MI 48178
Tel.: (800) 521-9746
(734) 769-5565
Fax: (734) 769-1708

Ocutech Vision Enhancement Systems
109 Connor Drive, Suite 2105
Chapel Hill, NC 27514
Tel.: (800) 326-6460
(919) 967-6460
Fax: (919) 967-8146
E-mail: info@ocutech
Web site: http://www.ocutech.com

Opteltec
36 Waltham Street
Lexington, MA 02193
Tel.: (617) 674-2499
Fax: (617) 674-2647

Sears Home Health Care Catalog
9804 Chartwell Drive
Dallas, TX
Tel.: (800) 326-1750

Programs and Technology

Integrated Visual Healing
655 Lewelling Boulevard, Suite 214
San Leandro, CA 94579

Tel.: (510) 357-0477
Web site: www.visualhealing.com

MicroStim Technology Incorporated
7881 Northwest Ninetieth Avenue
Tamarac, FL 33321
Tel.: (800) 326-9119
     (954) 720-4383
Fax: (954) 697-7984
Web site: www.microstim.com

National Center for Homeopathy
801 North Fairfax Street, Suite 306
Alexandria, VA 22314
Tel.: (703) 548-7790
Web site: www.homeopathic.org

School for Self-Healing
1718 Taraval Street
San Francisco, CA 94116
Tel.: (415) 665-9574
Fax: (415) 665-1318
Web site: www.self-healing.org

SUGGESTED READING

Bakker, R. *ElderDesign: Designing and Furnishing Your Home for Your Later Years.* New York: Penguin, 1997.

Berger, Jeffrey W., Stuart L. Fine, and Maureen G. Maguire. *Age-Related Macular Degeneration.* St. Louis: Mosby, 1999.

Grunwald, Henry. "Losing Sight." *New Yorker,* December 9, 1996, 62–67.

———. *Twilight: Losing Sight, Gaining Insight.* New York: Knopf, 1999.

Halloran, G. *Amazing Grace: Autobiography of a Survivor.* St. Cloud, Minn.: North Star, 1993.

Mogk, L., and Mogk. *Macular Degeneration: The Complete Guide to Saving and Maximizing Your Sight.* New York: Ballantine, 1999.

Retina Research Fund. *For My Patient: Macular Degeneration.* San Francisco: Retina Research Fund, 1997.

Rose, Marc R., M.D., and Michael R. Rose, M.D. *Save Your Sight! Natural Ways to Prevent and Reverse Macular Degeneration.* New York: Warner Books, 1998.

Sardi, B. *Nutrition and the Eyes.* Vol. 2. Montclair, N.J.: Health Spectrum, 1994.

Schneider, M. *Self-Healing. My Life and Vision.* London: ARKANA, Penguin, 1989.

Schneider, M., M. Larkin, and D. Schneider. *The Handbook of Self-Healing.* ARKANA, Penguin, 1994.

Silverman, B. *Bert's Eye View: Coping with Macular Degeneration.* Portland, Me.: Viewpoint Press, 1997.

Wason, B. *Macular Degeneration: Living Positively with Vision Loss.* Seattle: Hunter House, 1998.

INDEX